NOTES FOR HEALTHY KIDS

Amongst the world's most followed nutritionists, Rujuta Diwekar is a vocal champion of using our common sense and uncomplicating the act of eating.

Combining the latest in nutrition science with the traditional food wisdom from our homes, she advocates a multi-disciplinary approach towards our health. One that is devoid of fads and trends, which the food industry thrives on.

Her books have sold more than a million copies and continue to define the discourse on food and fitness across the country.

Notes for Healthy Kids

Rujuta Diwekar

First published by Westland Publications Private Limited in 2019

Published by Westland Books, a division of Nasadiya Technologies Private Limited, in 2022

No. 269/2B, First Floor, 'Irai Arul', Vimalraj Street, Nethaji Nagar, Alapakkam Main Road, Maduravoyal, Chennai 600095

Westland and the Westland logo are the trademarks of Nasadiya Technologies Private Limited, or its affiliates.

ISBN: 9789395073158

10 9 8 7 6

Typeset by Ram Das Lal, New Delhi, NCR

Printed at HT Media Ltd, Greater Noida

Contents

Introduction

i dream of a world where every child is free to play, learn and eat as she likes. If this dream is to be fulfilled, then every child should have access to good food. Food that nurtures and protects the tiny souls and sensitive hearts — and so, this book.

It is an attempt to knock some sense into parents, but then my editor asked me to not be so blunt. So here's how i will put it — the book is an attempt to keep our grandmothers' wisdom alive. The simple and uncomplicated way of living and eating. One of fun and masti, stories and fantasies, vacations and papad.

As the world gets global and 4G arrives on our phones, common sense seems to be packed off to a place so far that you would come across as a rebel if you even tried using it. On the other hand, constantly rubbing your hands with sanitiser would win approving glances. Eating and feeding young kids out of plastic containers with large cartoon characters is real, not stupid. And it is stupid to actually give your kids food in the silver thali that the grandmom so carefully chose from the limited options available.

'Everything, even change in behaviour, must be

packaged,' said my Berkeley-educated partner. i snorted in approval. Rarely do i agree on anything with anybody, least of all my partner. i hate the big school types, they bore me to death, but he did have a point.

Over the years, i have seen my clients, friends and even family torture their children over food, only to be tortured in return. What was once a joy and an expression of love has turned into a chore. It's like an accident: you don't remember how and what exactly happened but the damage is there for everyone to see. Similarly, we don't know when and exactly how, but tasteless foods with unpronounceable names and belonging to far-off places have gained a reputation for being healthy. It has nudged out simple, tasty and local foods like ghee-rice, banana-roti, etc. The damage here is the daily drama about food. It's tough to tell who the victim really is: the child or the parent. Both seem to be victimised, one bargaining for extra time on the iPad in exchange for finishing off the food on the plate, the other offering a packet of chips in return for eating two rotis. Now that's a spine-chilling barter, at least for me.

You don't know whether to speak or shut up; either way you are doomed. Much like the shaadi ka laddoo, damned if you do, damned if you don't. Why not a book then, which speaks to you when you are not in the heat of the moment. When you are not saying, drink this milk — it will make you grow taller; eat the dal — it is full of protein; finish your veggies — you need the greens, etc. One that tells you that you are not alone in this. That you have been systematically cultivated by the food and the weight loss industry, a trillion-dollar market today. It thrives on the fact that 'educated' means someone who has stopped listening to grandmother and has turned to Google for all research.

There you go, random people least interested in your well-being are now a more valuable resource and your mother's words just sound like a rant. 'Arre kuch nahi hota, give her some ghee-shakkar-roti', seems like an attempt to dislodge you from your heightened sense of what is good and bad food for your child. And from your Google rani status of a liberal, global citizen who believes that every child must be exposed to world cuisine, preferably rich in protein and good fats and low on carbs. Aaargh! No wonder then that your little one refuses to eat. She wants food, not nutrients. There, i said it. Food please, and not carbs, protein and fat in certain, specific proportions. Because by the time your kids grow up, that is going to be the wrong formula to eat; it will get replaced by something more complicated so that your kids feel even more intelligent and brave than you do when you urge them to chew on rucola and beet shreds. You will be left wondering where you went wrong. You will blame yourself for their illnesses, obesity, allergies. All this when all you fed them was 'healthy food'.

To cut a long story short, chillax. Food and eating is

bloody instinctive. Your child has a survival instinct and eating will come naturally. i will go to the extent of saying that eating sensibly will come naturally. The question is, will you allow it?

Happy reading and no more food shaming.

Rujuta Diwekar
Mumbai
December 2018

Part 1

The Bigger Picture

i hate being made to wait, but this was a CME (continuing medical education for doctors) and they invariably run late. In any case, i didn't have the time to debate in my head whether or not to leave without delivering my talk. The speaker on stage had gripped my attention and he was talking about parenting being an opportunity; specifically, four kinds of opportunities: the opportunity to create health, education, mistakes and technology, in that particular order.

Often, i have wondered how to describe a healthy child. Height and weight charts don't seem to do justice to the definition of health, nor does just being good in school or active in sports. But looking at parenting as an opportunity seemed to answer it for me — a healthy child is one who thrives in an environment of good food and love, goes to school, is allowed to make mistakes and has access to technology that is regulated by parents. The environment in which the child grows up also formed the basis of one of the largest studies ever undertaken by EU, the I.Family project. This was essentially to look at the factors that determine a child's susceptibility to obesity and non-communicable diseases, and then to come up with interventions that would lead to long-term healthy changes (more on this later).

Childhood obesity is now being looked at as a global public health crisis, which, if left unattended, unaddressed, could spell doom for our future and future generations. The problem is not so much about just being overweight but about the host of illnesses that it brings — diabetes, heart diseases, cancer, to a name a few — and the premature deaths and low quality of life that go with it. And while this is bad news, the good news is that all this is preventable. But for prevention, we have to look at children as a collective, as a public resource that all of us are responsible for. And know that parents are not solely responsible for the health of their children. We have to rise above our differences and as people, policymakers and governments, we must work together to ensure a healthy future for our children.

The health of your child is not just your responsibility

If our children are not unhealthy or overweight, it's a shocker — our green spaces are shrinking, our pollution levels are rising, big food giants are gunning for our kids with contests, ads, toys, and we still feel that it is either their personal failure or our parenting failure that they are fat. Relax, it's not.

For too long we have looked at obesity as what it is not — a personal problem brought about by a lack of will power, overeating or lazing around. When we subject children to this kind of understanding of health, we make things worse for them. A child doesn't get fat or unhealthy in isolation; all that you see in them is a representation of what is happening around them. *Bramhanda* to *pinda* and vice versa, as the Upanishads explain — all that you see in an individual is a reflection of all that there is in the universe or his environment. The fact is that we are raising children in an *obesogenic environment* — you could walk to school, your child is driven; you played downstairs for three hours every single day, your child doesn't or plays at the club maybe over the weekend; your mother made you hot nashta, your kid is eating cereal with milk or drinking juice or just going to school without food.

Being a parent today is riddled with challenges that were until recently unknown to mankind. i mean, when you and i were growing up, or even until fifteen years ago, if you did something wrong, you were at fault, not your parents. If you got hurt, if you got scolded in school, it was all your fault. Your parents called the shots, you suffered them — well, you know what i mean. If you came back saying that your friend is going to the US so even you want to go, your parents told you to go to hell. Today, they are looking at

EMI options for Miami Disney World. Other than your birthday or on the day you stood first in class or came home to announce that you were the school captain or till you were down with flu, no one at home did anything to please you. They loved you, yes. But no one serviced you. Everyone went on with their lives, and you were integrated into the eco-system — not vice versa.

But today, even if your child has a runny nose, it's your fault. There's something that you haven't done. Haven't refilled the sanitiser or given them a protein-rich diet or something. Children today, unfortunately, have been turned into consumers whose approval we must constantly seek. And yet, they are only tiny little beings who are entirely dependent on us. From sussu, to potty, from food to security, from schooling to recreation. In management classes, it is taught that the customer is not always right, and sometimes businesses have to tell customers what they want. In a way, i think that matches the definition of a healthy child. As a parent, you have the opportunity to create health, education, mistakes, technology — essentially, to define specifically what each one of them means for your child. Basically, you get to tell them what they want as food and exercise in order to have health, the primary need for a happy child.

Empowering, isn't it? And yet, today, as parents, empowered isn't exactly how we feel. The doc went on to give the example of one of his patients, a little eight-year-old boy who was brought to him by the parents, because they feared that he had an attention deficit problem. One of the boy's friends was shifting school because his parents were divorcing. The boy came home and asked his thirty-something father, 'What's a divorce?' The father came back home early the next Friday, took him to the Bandra family court, and gave him all the possible stats on divorce. How many happen every year, how many are initiated by women as compared to men, how different religions in India have different laws for divorces, etc. And then the father complained to the doc that, though he had done all he could to explain divorce to the child, the child seemed distracted, disinterested and even cranky at the Bandra court. All the child sought, explained the doc, was reassurance — 'Your mother and i are not divorcing, you will never have to change school'. Instead, he had received the most up-to-date information on divorce; that's not what he was seeking, and thus the lack of attention. We are complicating the smallest of issues because we want to be our kids' friends, not their parents. Being a parent is an opportunity; we must not let it pass. There's plenty of time to be friends later. For now, be a parent; lead, guide.

Scope of the Book

In India, we are facing a unique situation — we have the highest number of underweight and malnourished children in the world, the second-highest number of obese kids in the world, and let's not forget that we are also the diabetes capital of the world. While we have successfully brought down infant mortality and maternal deaths, we are still not fully equipped in our heads or in our policies to address the issues of obesity and non-communicable diseases that we are facing. Even at the government level, we feel that obesity is a marginal problem limited to the elite — it is not. As demographics shift, the underprivileged and poor are more exposed to obesity and its health and economic costs; the rural to urban migration makes previously malnourished kids obese quickly, but the underlying issues of malnourishment or under-nutrition continue.

And while i hope that our policymakers and governments take note of the fact that childhood obesity is not a lifestyle issue but brought about by political and policy failure, it's imperative that we as people and parents do not reduce it to a carbohydrate, protein, fat, calorie, portion-size problem. Seeing the issue as it exists is step one to addressing it, wouldn't you agree? That doesn't make food- and nutrition-related conversation completely useless for our children's health, but in fact more relevant than before.

So for now and in the scope of this book, we will focus on good nutrition (and also exercise and sleep) and how it affects the quality of our life. It will be about how food can be used effectively to lay down the foundation of growth, development and sustainable health and well-being for our children. And to acknowledge that health is the only thing that we owe them. And that if we have passed down the means of earning health, then, with their efforts, exposure and expertise, they can earn and enjoy all the wealth they want.

PART 1a: FOOD

Chapter 1

For Parents — Beyond Food Confusion

The food confusion

Food — it really should have been the simplest thing in the world, but we have complicated it to such an extent that, even when you are doing something as innocent as drinking water, you are not sure whether or not you are doing it right. Should it be before food or after? Bottled or RO? But even then, food remains one of our natural instincts; eating is one of the first acts that we perform upon taking birth. Food soothes a crying baby, helps build the connection to the mother, sustains life, lays the foundation to growth, development, maturity, nurtures the body, mind, spirit, and without it, life itself would not be possible.

Annaad bhootani jayante, say the Upanishads; it's through food that all living beings take birth and grow.

Adyate atti cha bhootaani, tasmaad annam taduchyate iti. That which is consumed by human beings and consumes them in turn is anna. Deep, isn't it, and so true, especially in our modern, fast-paced and information-overloaded lives. Parenting, then, means teaching our children to eat in a way in which food doesn't consume them. Childhood is the best time to teach them the right values of food and to future-proof their health. A healthy childhood gives birth to a healthy adolescence and a healthy, mature adult. Think about it more like a fifty-year return on investment.

UNITED NATIONS' SUSTAINABLE DEVELOPMENT GOALS

Our scriptures teach us that anna is the route to ananda, the true nature of human beings. If this is the timeless teaching of any native culture, the seventeen UN's SDGs too are in tune with it. Two out of the top three goals are related to food, health and well-being for all. Good nutrition as the driver of the seventeen SDGs and development beyond just GDP or economic aspects is the global aspiration for the future. It's about nutritious food, gender equality, water and sanitation, rights of indigenous people, sustainable cities, clean air, responsible production and consumption, life on land and below water, peace, justice, strong institutions, etc. Without a more equal and equitable world, economic prosperity or growth will mean nothing. Food, the way we grow it, how we store it, the way we consume it, are all foundations to a better world, and a happy, harmonious world order.

Parenting turns into a joy when children are allowed to be their natural selves. And when they are not, you have a picky, fussy, frequently ill version of a perfectly healthy child. Letting a child be is an act of extreme courage. Because it's an act of letting go. And almost nothing is as binding as the attachment to a child. From attachment comes fear. Fear that somehow we are not good enough parents, that somehow we are not feeding them enough protein or calcium or even vitamins, fear that we are depriving them of a good life. And fear, you must remember, is the opposite of love and good health. For parenting to remain an opportunity to create good health, it must confront fear, and the only way to do that is with facts. Vidya can only come to those who have experienced avidya, observe our scriptures. Courage is not the absence of fear but the ability to overcome it, is the pop version of the same thing.

What created the food confusion

Many things, but these two phenomena are primarily responsible for the food confusion and misinformation we are dealing with today.

1. Nutrition transition

In 1993, food science researcher Barry Popkin proposed a framework called nutrition transition — 'the transition of traditional eating patterns to Western pattern diets'. Western diet here stands for food that is more processed and packaged. It applies to countries like ours and even to China, Brazil — basically every country that gets called as 'developing'. As our population gets more global and urban, we move less and less, our physical activity drops, and we eat differently from what we have done traditionally. To realise how nutrition transition works in daily life, consider this: It's a weekend and you make pancakes or crêpes for your kids, as a treat. Or, it's your kid's birthday and you are throwing a party at the food hall of a mall, where his friends get treated to burgers and feel happy. Or, you open your refrigerator and there's a soda bottle or fruit-flavoured drink cooling its heels in one of the compartments. Or, your husband is cooking tonight, and he has whipped up an amazing spaghetti aglio e olio and not khichdi.

If one or all of them apply to you, then you are already a part of nutrition transition. Your kids are currently eating very differently from the way their grandparents or even you ate at their age. And, according to research, this puts them at a high risk of developing NCDs, that's non-communicable diseases: diabetes, heart disease, obesity, cancer, mental health issues, etc. It happens over a period of time, and with long-term exposure. So, a pancake or soda over an odd weekend won't do it, but if you have it week after week, month after month, year after year, well, now the risk is real. Get it?

Nutrition transition happens primarily because of two reasons:

- Lack of value of native foods.
- Intelligent food marketing and positioning by food industry.

Native foods and eating habits are such an intrinsic part of daily life that our foremothers thought it inappropriate to link every food to a specific nutrient and then to a perceived benefit. *Tadeva brahma-twam viddhi nedam yadi-damupaasate*, goes a line from the Upanishads. It broadly means: that which appears as God or reality is not quite the God or reality. Applying this wisdom to food reality, carrots may appear to be a source of vitamin A, but without adequate fat in the diet, the vitamin A or whatever little vitamin A is present in the carrot will be unavailable or malabsorbed by the body. Instead, pumpkin, a native, low-profile vegetable, in the form of kaddu ka sabzi or a bhopala bharit (kaddu ka raita), gives a much better chance for the body to assimilate the carotene (a form of vitamin A), as it already comes with the essential fat and spices and herbs that act as co-factors in converting carotene to vitamin A (usable form) in the body. Now since our grandmoms were aware of this reality, they thought of kaddu ka sabzi or bhopala bharit as delicacies to be enjoyed at certain times of the year, especially during certain festivals and fasts. Kaddu cooked the right way is much more than vitamin A, after all, and the primary function of food is to provide joy, nourishment and protection.

WHEN ASPIRATION HURTS

If i was to point out the one thing that stands in the way of our children and their optimum health, then i would say it's aspiration. With a capital A. Aspiration to be more global and its portrayal as being that which is divorced from all that is native and local. With real estate, cars, mobile phones, it's all ok, it's maaf, because these don't enter inside your stomach and become a part of you (though they influence what you will allow inside your mouth), but with food, it's a complete game-changer. You get what i am saying? You change Dariya Mahal with fourteen coconut trees to Fioranza with fifteen floors, all-glass façade, only palm trees like in Singapore, and you have already lost a lot on identity, your environment, your birds, bees, flowers; everything just got poorer, but you are feeling rich. i get that. (Actually, i don't.) But when you do this with food, when poha is switched with oats, paratha with Chocos, banana with juice, you get, you get, well, you get a raw deal. You just switched from rich food to poor food, and it made your child's health so poor that the most expensive medicine and healthcare won't be able to cure it. The cure here lies in prevention. You have to simply prevent this transition from rich food to poor food.

2. *Nutritionism*

If food or anna has to lead to ananda, or to the SDGs for 2030, which aim to end poverty, protect the planet and ensure prosperity for all in the next ten–twelve years, then it must expand itself beyond the caged view of carbohydrate, protein and fat. Looking at food from the point of view of nutrients is called as nutritionism (coined by author and activist, Michael Pollan); it reduces food to what it is not. Like all other isms — racism, sexism, ageism — it misses out on the bigger picture and leads to decisions being made on the basis of biases and fears, not facts. We must be able to see food in the way the future beckons us to see it, from a multidisciplinary approach. One which encourages you to take into consideration a much wider, expanded, real view, deliberating on things that didn't even cross your mind earlier, pretty much like the definition of parenthood. Now that the child is involved, her well-being, safety, security, success in the future is involved, everything takes a new shape, a new definition, a new view. Similarly, the expanded and real view of food must include things like crop cycle, soil health, land use, agriculture policies, farmer welfare, local economy, global ecology, climate change, gender equality and much more. This is called the 'Food system' view as against the 'Food group' view of nutritionism.

In 2012, in Newcastle, UK, sitting in the audience listening to a panel comprising mostly nutrition academicians, i heard candid admissions about how the whole idea of looking at food from the reductionist view of carbohydrate, protein, fat had backfired. Instead of helping the public make better decisions about food, it had helped the food industry (which doesn't need to be helped by universities). They talked about how the common man was more confused than ever about the smallest things like bread. To eat or not to eat, to gluten or not to gluten, they said to a giggling audience. In 2015, at the FENS conference in Berlin, similar admissions were made about how scientific outcomes related to food and nutrition had doubled in the last five years, but not the number of scientists, clearly pointing to the poor quality of nutrition studies and researches done. And about the unfortunate nexus between the food industry, researchers and mainstream media.

Globally, diets are getting more like each other, and fading in quality, diversity and health outcomes. NCDs alone are projected to cost the world 47 trillion US dollars in the next two decades. And with that we have the double burden of malnourishment — underweight, overweight — and now the new category of micronutrient-deficient (e.g. vitamin D, B12, Fe) people across the globe. The thing about double burden, or as it is now called, triple burden of malnourishment, is that it is characterised by the prevalence of underweight, overweight and diet-related lifestyle diseases, within the same person, same household and same populations. Developing countries like ours are witnessing a 30 per cent faster rise in overweight and obese children as compared to richer nations. And while India continues to have a high number of child mortality deaths due to diarrhoea (lack of sanitation, hygiene), kids from affluent families are developing allergies, infections and intolerances akin to the Western, sanitised / sterilised world.

So what does this mean for the health and well-being of our children? Everything. Nutrition transition and nutritionism work hand-in-hand, and they have only one agenda — profits, not public health. If the East India Company came through the trade route, the food industry is coming through the nutrient route. Nutritionism tells us to eat nutrients, not food, and nutrition transition makes us feel our local produce is 'not good enough' and gives us 'better alternatives'. Want fibre? Eat oats, not banana. Want good fat? Cook with olive oil, not filtered ground nut oil. Want protein? Eat soya, not legumes.

The best thing is that they never explicitly tell you what not to eat. Ditch the local is implied here, not instructed. This is soft colonisation; it leaves you poorer and denies you your right to your unique identity, your regional recipes, and as we are discovering now, even gut-friendly microbes. The food industry doesn't just send these messages to you through mainstream media, celeb endorsements or by influencing government policies; their shackles are deep into our education system too. When i did my post-graduation in sports science and nutrition, i only studied food through the prism of food groups, calorie counting and portion sizes. It was like nothing else existed or mattered. A lot of our food beliefs now come out of that. A lot of what we believe is food science is what we have been taught to see; this isn't science though, it's nutritionism. Science, as we know it, is all encompassing; it looks at the smallest thing from the widest possible angle.

STUDYING NUTRITION IN INDIA

Scientific understanding of food would mean, first of all, studying where it's coming from. But farmers and farming find no mention in the textbooks of nutrition colleges. Culture, crop cycles, climate, practices, preparation, fairs, festivals, community — these are things that we should be studying. Also soil health, native species, change of land use, depleting water sources, GMOs, food policies, MSP. But no, there isn't a word, a lecture, or even a thought about these things. Region, religion, rituals, even these influence food and food beliefs, but again there is no mention of them. The narrative is only and only around nutrients and calorie counts. Cereal companies sponsor competitions, yogurt companies give out T-shirts, juice companies give you free trials and no one blinks, much less screams 'conflict of interest!'. Well, to be fair, all syllabi need a major upgrade, but because food and nutrition is what our life, our health, our well-being depend on, this is one area that is sacred. And this should be protected from vested interests. The reason why i often think that nutritionists and dietitians are not as smart as they think they are is because they never question

> what they have learnt. They must, if they must serve people. If you don't unlearn, you serve profits. And that's a loss-making proposition in the long run.

Clearing the Food Confusion

Sometimes, it can all be quite overwhelming, but the truth is that the answer to the most complicated problems of the world is often simple. This is absolutely true about food and nutrition. For centuries, men and women ate what grew around them, ate it fresh and in season, and felt grateful for what was on their plate. They believed that food was a resource that must not be wasted or abused. They shared what they had, stored what they could — grains and pulses — and fermented / pickled other perishables for future use. If you download the UN SDG document to check out what you can do individually, at home and at work, to save the world, you will pretty much find the same grandmom wisdom there. Switch off lights when you don't need them, buy local food produce that doesn't involve trucks and planes to land on your plate, air dry your clothes and hair, etc. It seems so silly and small, you will feel that this is not going to help. But it is really like how you build fitness: it's not about that one workout, it's about that one workout that you do five times a week over five years, and what you see and enjoy is the compounding, cumulative effect.

Our children will be living in challenging times — AI, climate change, wars over water and food, and god knows what else. But if they have inherited the right food values from us, then they will learn to lead meaningful, fulfilling, purposeful lives. One where their main aim in life won't be to knock off 5 kg by December or to fit into size 4 for a wedding, but to be free. Free to define health, wealth and happiness for themselves. By 2050, we will be a global population of almost ten billion people, and hunger will be one of the major issues then, as will be the deaths and disabilities due to non-communicable diseases. We have about thirty years to get our act together; let's start from anna, because anna is the route to ananda.

So here are the **four food fundas for parents,** condensed into easy-to-understand facts and fears:

i. *Fact: Local, seasonal and traditional food is good for you*
   Fear: Food that has proteins, fats and carbs in a certain ratio is good for you

Before we go ahead, let me just clarify that food as a sum total of carbs, protein, fat and calories is unscientific and entirely industry driven. We are systematically made to look at our diets as carbs, protein, fat and calories through influencers, health professionals and mainstream media. The whole idea is to subtly and not so subtly discredit local foods, portray them as insufficient in one or more nutrients and to offer healthier alternatives in the form of industrialised food products. Before we know it, the fear that our home-grown food is somehow lacking in essential nutrients has consumed us all and in turn allowed food companies to employ us as its consumers. This only helps profits and not people, you know that by now.

Our grandmothers never asked us to eat anything because it was rich in one nutrient or the other. Instead, they introduced us to the rich tradition of eating something because it is in season, they patronised local produce long before it became fashionable to do so. Actually, our aajis, dadis, nanis, pattis are the original global citizens.

Mine said things like, *Shastra mhanun kha;* eat because that's the science. She said this to me when she asked me to add ghee to my puran poli. i told her she was just a ball of superstition. She instantly forgave me, i don't think she even minded; she just smiled and poured the ghee. Years later, i learnt, well after my post-graduation in sports science and nutrition, that ghee was and is a fat burner. It leads to better assimilation of vitamin D and all fat-soluble vitamins, is essential to maintain the diversity and number of gut-friendly bacteria, leads to a better blood sugar response, etc. But from the 1970s–2000, until even later, it was banned by the very people we trusted would know science — doctors mainly and dietitians who sang along, and mainstream media articles. When i said to her that she was a ball of superstition, i was only ten and my school hadn't officially taught me about carbs, protein and fat, but i was already aware of the 'dangers' of saturated fat. Just like that, kids get the drift of what society considers scientific and backward and everything in between.

Well, i was a kid and my stupidity was instantly forgiven and ignored by Mamai (that's what i called her; she was my neighbour and looked after me while my mom kept her job as a lecturer of organic chemistry), but it is not quite as simple when it is kids who are at the receiving end. The wife of one of my clients told me that her eight-year-old likes instant noodles a lot and it's cool because it's very healthy. i must have looked confused, because she went on to explain that it was oats noodles and that too she made it with tons of veggies. And that i should wipe that expression off my face because she was not so stupid that she would just offer a small kid regular maida noodles. Actually, on most days, i have a pretty cool job, one where i can speak my mind. But every now and then, there are moments like this, where i raise my eyebrows and try hard to give an approving smile but it doesn't always work out, you know. This one ended with the woman telling me that she better not see this in my next book. Some other versions of the same story are — ragi for packaged cereal, kiwi for immunity, or formula as weaning-off food instead of rice porridge.

Basically, the question we need to ask ourselves is: am i adopting a new food or banning an old food (that's part of my food heritage) on the basis of advice that is nutrient based? The 'iss mein protein hai, iron hai, fibre hai, etc.', formula? And if i am, then both the person who is giving me that advice and i for taking it have been played by the food industry. Not only do big food companies make money out of us, but the constant propaganda of choosing foods based on nutrients leaves us in a constant state of fear. The fear that we may not be getting adequate amounts of x or y nutrient for our optimal health. It takes the fun away from traditions and leaves us in a state of confusion for years to come. Food and traditions are meant to infuse confidence, the type that comes from feeling light and content post a meal. The type that allows us to come around to the fact that, just like money doesn't buy happiness, nutrients don't buy health — it all boils down to striking that right balance in life. To be able to enjoy food but not be consumed by it. Eating simple, home-cooked meals with local ingredients that are in season and cooked as per tradition is a time-tested way of getting there.

GHEE

India, the land of ghee, first switched to refined vegetable oils about forty years ago, and then to virgin olive oil in the last decade. Then, in September

2016, Cleveland Clinic in the US, where all rich Indians go for a bypass, released a poster on ghee and its many benefits for human health. And now it's routine for you to get ghee or clarified butter in supermarket stores in the West. But between all this, we forgot that science is exact and precise by its very nature; it is also broadminded. If ghee was not ok in the 1970s, if it led to heart diseases in the 1980s, diabetes in the 1990s, then it can't be the answer to all human health problems in 2016. And if that is the cycle it has gone through, it's not food science, it's food business. Food science is ghee being one of the panch amrits in India for centuries together and valued for its benefits by one and all. The medical community finally accepting its scientific validity in 2016 is ok, that's allowed. That happens. What should not happen is native communities like ours giving up on everything traditional, indigenous, part of our food heritage in the name of science or some nutrient. Ghee, coconut, rice, sugarcane, everything seems to be going through this cycle. Coconut is now THE oil in the West, rice konjee is sold as veg protein in downtown Manhattan, and yes, you get sugarcane juice for a cleanse in San Francisco. Native communities are put off their own food, so that a market is created to turn their food products into a lucrative business.

Forty years for us to discover the truth while it is so easily available in our kitchens, is just a poor show of confidence by all of us. Let our kids inherit better.

ii. *Fact: Eating is a natural act and appetite is a moving entity*
Fear: A child must be tempted / coerced into eating and finishing a fixed quantity of food

If your household is the type where the only time the child directly accesses food is when it's laid on the table, then expect drama over everything. And i don't just mean the fuss that the child will throw at bhendi being cooked instead of aloo, but also the one that you will throw. Where you will worry that they are not eating enough or make statements like, really Rujuta, i am telling you, maybe you won't believe me, but my child can really go for days without eating. So how many days is that? No one has the answer to that because the reality is that the child is just threatening to not eat every day. Then the mother is incentivising the act of finishing everything on the plate by offering extra iPad time or a chocolate or some other equally random but unhealthy thing. So if the child is always unhappy with what's being cooked, and if you are always fussing over how little he's eating, it's just an environment where value for food is missing. The good news is that can change the moment you decide to involve the kids in the kitchen.

KITCHEN AND KIDS

No matter whether you are rich or poor, man or woman, have staff or no staff, enter the kitchen and have your kids help you lay the food on the table. Ok, ok, if not on all days, most days. If not at all meals, most meals; at least one meal a day, do this. Children will not learn to appreciate what's on their plate if they are completely disconnected with the process of what all it takes for the food to land on your plate. The kitchen is the easiest place to start from. Start there and take the inconvenience in your stride.

Have them pick up their plates and clean up the table after, as well — regardless of gender or age group. And before you roll your eyes at the difficulty of this task, know that kids across the globe do this, it's really not a biggie. Humare Indian bachhe hi nahi karte, because parents nahi karte. You know, when children are really small, they want to sweep the floor, swab it, and do saaf-safai as a game, because activity is really attractive and natural to children. Then, over time, they realise that they are growing up in a feudal environment or that it's not cool to do your own tasks yourself. Basically, they learn organically that you shouldn't move your body much if you are rich enough to pay someone else to do things for you. And over a period of time, the attraction to be active fades away, and it gets replaced by entitlement. Unknowingly, we have laid the foundation to unhappiness and sickness right there.

But this is a bit like getting out of shape physically — it's reversible if you are patient with yourself and take the approach of one step at a time. You have to create that culture of value for food, and everyone must participate in the kitchen.

In no time, you will see that they are eating better, slower and are happier with everything that's on the plate; that's the power of ownership. Now it's food that they laid on the table, they helped cook and serve, now they will eat it with pride. It's like how Indian mothers feel that their sons are better than every boy on earth — ownership. Ideally, we should teach our children a bit of farming too, and take them to farms often; but that may not always be possible. The kitchen is taking them a step closer to the farm; once they see and experience the labour that goes into making meals, there is almost no chance of a fuss. And if there ever is, you can attribute it to hunger; quickly get them to eat so that they get over it. Banana is the handiest, easiest and fastest-acting medicine for hunger, btw.

The other thing that you must know is that it is pretty natural for the appetite to fluctuate. It changes according to the season, vacation, school, stress — everything. Encourage your children to respect their appetites, serve accordingly and ask them to chew their meal slowly. In the meantime, you also get off the phone or whatever else you are on and watch how they eat; better still, eat along with them. How they eat and how much they are eating will give you good insight into what they are feeling; dull and slow or happy and energetic. If you fix a magical quantity in your head — you can't get up before eating two rotis, etc. — then you have opened yourself to drama.

Childhood is a powerless state, one where you have no vocabulary to explain that — 1) In summer my appetite naturally dips 2) i had a tough game, i am slightly pukey right now, i can't eat it all 3) It's winter, my appetite is up 4) My fav cousin is here, my appetite is enlarged: shared laughter, shared food 5) Hmm, it's my favourite meal, i can eat endlessly 6) Can't eat, plain dehydrated, give me some water first, then give me food and i will eat, etc. Parenting, however, is that unaccountable powerful state where, if you wish, you can interpret what's happening and help the child nourish herself.

In real life, however, kids know that the best way to get out of this powerless state is manipulation. They use it to their advantage to make you feel at a serious disadvantage. Of course, this only happens if you have fixed a quantity and are fussing that they are not eating enough. Then, they will manipulate you in one of various ways (all are not covered here): 1) Will eat only if you give them ketchup with it 2) iPad or extra video game time for finishing the meal 3) Only if you give them a chocolate / ice cream at the end of the meal 4) Throwing away the plate or generally creating a ruckus 5) Howling, sobbing, not talking, etc. If you see any of these things happening, *relex,* as they would say in Gujarat; know that you are the powerful one, that you are bigger than your child's drama (affirmation). And tell them, softly, tumko dukh nahi, bhukh laga hai. No problem, anytime you are ready, you have this tasty, fresh meal. You will get nothing else to eat, it's your responsibility to eat, you are a big, strong girl / boy. Jitna khane ka hai, utna hi khao, no pressure on quantity. i will eat with you, ok? Come, let's eat. Soft in your words, stable and firm in your conduct, that's how Mamai was; model yourself after her. She raised four granddaughters, and we all turned out healthy, with a good body image and we never fell for a crash diet — it's no mean feat. But you have to be like her: persistent, gentle; give the kids no leeway when it comes to common sense and food values. Go for it momma, i am with you.

iii. *Fact: Sit, switch off, senses — the three S's of eating right*

Fear: Eating is important, not how

Who wouldn't like to raise a child who is not deficient in micronutrients like vitamin D and B12, has high bone mineral density and a flat stomach? But then, for that, we have to adopt our food heritage in its full glory. The only way local, seasonal and traditional meals work is when you have digested them, assimilated and absorbed all the goodness they have to offer and excreted all the by-products. Your posture while eating, then, is of paramount importance; basically, you have to optimise blood flow to the stomach to ensure that digestion is taking place optimally.

According to Ayurveda, less than optimal digestion is the foundation of every known and unknown disease. Falling sick every season change, constipation, irritability, are just some of the obvious signs of indigestion. Drop in friendly gut bacterial diversity, inability to assimilate vitamin B12 and D, getting too tired too quickly, painful periods are some more telling signs. As are as acne, dependence on stimulants like coffee or Red Bulls, and inability to fall asleep. Basically, every age group has its own unique version of this less-than-optimum digestion. The solution is so simple that you may be tempted to discard it instantly, but i am gonna try nevertheless.

The three S's of eating right:

1. *Sit:* First of all, sitting on the floor with our legs in sukhasana, cross-legged, is amongst the best therapies for our joints. The spine learns to align itself, the muscles of the back learn to engage themselves, the pelvic joint learns to open — it's like stability, strength and stretching in just one go. No wonder then that it's also the preferred position for prayer, worship and meditation too. A stable spine means — no paunch and optimum height growth. Strong muscles mean — good posture, better strength in athletic performance. A flexible pelvic joint means — better oxygenation to the testes / ovaries and vagina, quick recovery from sports performance, less chance of falling and pulling or breaking anything in the body. And, of course, sitting cross-legged directs the flow of blood to the stomach, leading to optimum digestion. So more than one reason to sit in sukhasana. All Asian, Middle-Eastern and African cultures sit on the floor and eat; it's nothing to be ashamed or embarrassed about. You can use it to your advantage, in fact, like the Korean restaurants on 32nd Street in New York, which use 'sit and eat' as one of their USPs, and find takers amongst the young, affluent and cool kids. So, yes, get your

child off that high chair and encourage her to sit on the ground and eat.

2. *Switch off:* Get off the gadgets, of all kinds, whether it's the phone, iPad or TV, ideally forever but definitely while eating. Munching while viewing is not just scientifically linked to obesity, but even stereotypically, every cartoon of a fat person has him perched in front of a TV set. If you go by the I.Family study: a) Just having a TV in the kid's bedroom is a cardio-metabolic risk for the future. b) Children who watch TV during meals demand and drink more sugar-sweetened beverages (colas, caffeinated drinks and chocolate shakes, even juices), and are therefore at a further risk of developing obesity and related NCDs. c) Girls are at a higher risk of developing a negative body image with TV viewing during mealtimes. d) Excess TV viewing is linked to family dysfunction.

   So how much gadget time per day? Not more than thirty minutes (excluding homework and assignments on the laptop, if any), and not while eating.

   The underlying cause of gadget use during mealtimes is often fact 2 above — trying every trick in the trade to get the child to eat and then obsessing about quantities that itna nahi khaya toh grow kaise hoyega. But please, this really does need to stop. Mealtimes are for nourishment, not for entertainment, and digestion is affected by distraction. And eating together strengthens the bond between family members; it brings people together. It is not a task that you should quickly get off the list so you can post the next update, samjha kya?

3. *Senses:* Basically, count what is within and not outside. A life lesson served so matter-of-factly and simply by our food heritage that we may forget its significance to our adult life. Watch the food and nothing else, eat with hands, smell the aroma, chew slowly so that you can hear yourself eating and let the tongue guide you with the perception of taste. Hmm, just focus on food, said many a grandma, and almost all have indulgently scolded you when you declared how many puran polis, modaks or pooris you ate. 'Don't count how much you have eaten, just eat as much as you need.' Keeping all your senses focused on food helped you nurture your appetite, eat as per the need or hunger and, most importantly, allowed kids to self-terminate the act of eating.
   Physiologically, it meant that leptin, a hormone that signals that you are full and helps you stay calm (and in charge of your quantities), remained sensitive. Leptin resistance, like insulin resistance, is one of the known factors for obesity and NCDs. Psychologically, listening to the leptin signal and terminating the act of eating by itself made you feel empowered, like you were adulting. The fact that you got that right meant that you didn't need a smarter adult, app or professional to help with the basic task of eating; you could do it yourself. It's like

being able to do everything related to potty yourself, a coming of age in many ways. On a more spiritual note, it constantly rang home the message that it's about receiving more from less. Not about consuming more, but receiving more, sharing more. It put you in a happy mode and that was the default setting. A subtle message of 'don't waste your time on the outside, focus inside', delivered so sweetly that you had all the time on earth to chew on it. The exact opposite message is sent when we focus on the outside and tell kids that they won't be strong or tall or energetic if they don't consume everything on the plate, a foundation for unsteadiness and inadequacies, sadly.

iv. Fact: No variety for dinner and finish by 8 p.m.

Fear: Have to keep dinners interesting so that my child eats.

i can never say this enough, but the kuch khata nahi hai, sirf noodles khata hai kind of episodes should be stopped from playing themselves out. And it's easy to do that if you put your foot down. The I.Family study confirms what our culture always knew. Saying 'no' to kids when they are demanding unhealthy stuff and being unreasonable protects them from developing cardio-metabolic risks in the future. That's obesity and the NCDs that come with it. We want our children to grow up strong, resilient, happy, and for that to happen, we must raise them in the right food environment.

Cooking hajjar, ok five varieties for dinner means: i) You have a BIG fridge, your ingredients are never fresh, and ii) You have people with NCDs at home already. If you don't want your child growing up with an NCD, then for that, they have to wait for their turn of favourite food to come. Learning to eat someone else's favourite sabzi some nights is not a bad deal at all because a) it brings immense pleasure when yours is cooked b) you learn how to live with other people without complaining c) you discover what other things you can eat with rice or roti if you don't want to eat the dal or sabzi — e.g. achaar or ghee and namak or ghee and jaggery. A child who can be creative with food and improvise with what's available will find joy in every small aspect of life. Isn't that what you want?

And yes, if you must eat chaat or pav bhaji or some exotic stuff like khow suey and the likes, keep it for once in a while and have it in the evening between 4 and 6 p.m. and teach your kids to eat it in a way that still allows them to have khichdi or dahi-rice or a glass of milk by 8-ish.

The right food environment is not about avoiding sugar, scampering for protein or fussing over hygiene, but really about knowing where the gaps in our real food environment lie. Typically, in urban India, children eat really late; i wouldn't be off the mark if i said 9 or 9.30 p.m. is when most city kids will have dinner. This is what we need to focus on — that we feed our children so late; instead, we really focus on the non-essentials, thanks to the food confusion. Then, the fact is that they will eat in front of a gadget, you already know that that's wrong, so i won't repeat myself. Instead i will tell you something i haven't told you yet.

Kids who eat 'boring' dinners, and eat them early, grow the fastest and stay the strongest. Because it allows them to optimise on the non-negotiable and underrated aspect of good health — good sleep. Late meals mean late bedtime, which means that sleep is going to be compromised. If sleep was not important, evolution would have discarded it just like it discarded the tail. But it didn't. Mother nature is wise and she knows that, without good sleep, little children will not grow to their full potential — be it mentally, physically or sexually. That's why she gives out signals to parents so they may use their good sense and intervene. Allergies, intolerances, constipation, frequent illnesses, poor performance in school, anger, crankiness, withdrawal — look closely at their sleep pattern, especially the teenagers and under-fives, and take quick steps to correct it.

SCOLDED BY RATAN TATA

i was flying business class on a Singapore–Mumbai flight (using miles, please note) and seated right behind me was a guy who seemed to be on a diet of some kind. He first called for popcorn (popcorn, alcohol, chocolate, coffee is allowed on all diets, please note) and then complained that there were only fourteen pieces of popcorn in the box he had been offered. He was a middle-aged guy with the temperament of a cranky teen; the air hostesses, one after the other, were trying to cheer him up. 'Let me get you one more box,' i heard one of them say. Then, after the meal was served, he was unhappy with the dessert and wanted a sugar-free chocolate mousse instead. The air hostess offered a sugar-free ice cream they had on board, but he wanted mousse. 'Please sir, let us bring a smile on your face. May i offer you our 90 per cent dark chocolate?' Ahh, i couldn't take it anymore and i got up from my seat and went to the only place on an aircraft where you can find privacy — the loo. When i came out, the lady who was willing to do anything to put a smile on the gentleman's face was standing by the counter.

'Oh come on,' i said to her, almost involuntarily. 'When are you going to tell him off? You girls do such great work, but our collective pride as working women is at risk here if you continue to do all you can to put a smile on his face while the rest of your well-behaved guests get ignored.'

The air hostess smiled nervously and told me that yes, i was right. 'You know ma'am, once we had the pleasure of flying Mr Ratan Tata on our flight and there was a similar guest. He was standing here and arguing with us when Mr Tata got out of the loo. "Let me remind you young man," said Mr Tata, "this is not a restaurant, it's a flight." "Oh, i am sorry Mr Tata, i didn't mean to disturb you." "i am not," said Mr Tata, "i am just sorry for the people who have to live with you every day."'

What a brutal take-down, woh bhi kiske haath. The next time you are fussing over your little one and pleading, beta ji, kya khaoge, chalo aap ke liye mamma kya banaye, just know that sitting miles away from you, Tata ji is feeling sorry for you.

Top three misconceptions about food that parents have

In any school that i go to, when i tell kids that i am writing a book for them and it's going to tackle three main things: 1) Why you don't need to eat dal to get protein 2) Why you don't need to drink milk to get calcium 3) Why you don't need to eat vegetables to get your vitamins, i see fists thumping in the air, dabs and floss. We have made the instinctive, intelligent, intuitive act of eating food into a chore for future generations. But it doesn't need to be like this.

Let's look at these three misconceptions about food that have tortured almost every Indian child:

1. Milk for calcium

Being a parent is tough but gulping a glass of milk with someone staring at you is even tougher. And no, it doesn't get any easier because someone kisses you at the end or says mera achha bachha. In fact, schools now teach that there is a word for it — it's called manipulation. Manipulation happens when you don't know any better. Is calcium important for health, height and bones? Yes. Is it critical to get calcium only from milk? No. Are there other sources from which you can get calcium? Yes. So is it ok to not drink milk, like ever? Yes.

There are many sources of calcium that kids have absolutely no problems consuming. Til chiki, besan ladoo, ragi kheer or dosa, for example, but the problem is that we have not been trained to see them as sources of calcium. Even a handful of nuts, sundals or usal or misals, idli sambar with drumsticks, etc., are good sources. As are the many native and local veggies that are eaten specifically on certain festivals or are available only in specific seasons. But we don't see them as calcium sources because Indian food heritage is not boring. It's expansive enough to know that food provides multiple nutrients, feelings and benefits; to link it to one nutrient is a disservice. The other disservice is to feed them 'milk' from non-dairy sources like almond, etc., to make up for calcium. You really don't need to do that.

Basically, like love, you will find calcium in places where you are not looking. Two big, but unknown, sources of calcium, are:

i. Ragi: known to be Hanuman's favourite food. Hanuman is celebrated for his power and strength, and both come from good bone mineral density, specially the ability to carry heavy stuff. Remember the story of Hanuman carrying the mountain? So one can easily carry or, as is depicted, fly while carrying things heavier than one's body weight when one is strong in bone mineral density. Chalo, make ragi a weekly habit now — laddoo, dosa, porridge, or just roll it into a roti.

ii. Moringa: i am sure you have eaten sambar and found a drumstick in it. Now drumstick ka cool name is moringa, and recently, at a course i studied in Germany, it's been identified and looked up to as 'future food'. Future food is about foods that are resilient and will survive climate change and continue to provide taste and nourishment for the ever-increasing population on earth.

What you should totally avoid: mixing sugar powders parading around as protein drinks or health drinks in milk to kill the taste and smell of milk. It's pretty simple — you don't like milk, you don't drink milk, at least not for calcium.

But there's stuff that you can add that won't mask the taste, is natural and safe for you and is even a good source of calcium. E.g., badam, cashew, pista powder, saffron. Only valid if the kid likes milk in the first place.

Important note: Calcium absorption

The key to calcium absorption and assimilation is activity and exercise. We should be teaching this in school — that daily outdoor playing is what builds strong bones, not calcium. Without sports, outdoor games and activity, it's impossible for the body to get the stimuli required to build strong bones. So what is critical here is sport and games, not milk.

2. Dal for protein

This is one of my least favourites. Often said by parents who also tend to say things like, yeh kuch nahi khata. i mean, first of all, stop the exaggeration. If your child is really not eating anything, how is she going about her daily life? The thing is that we make children victims of our nutritionism. Is there protein in dal? Yes. Is it the only source of protein? Darn, no. Will your child be denied protein just because she doesn't like dal? No, nahi, kabhi nahi.

Now see, most kids till about two years of age are quite non-fussy about eating dal with their chawal (usually dal is pre-soaked before cooking and also made very diluted or watery for them). Then somewhere from about two-and-a-half till six–seven years of age, some kids go through a phase where they develop a natural aversion to dal. The reason is that dals naturally contain an anti-nutrient called 'trypsin and chymotrypsin inhibitor'. Trypsin and chymotrypsin are enzymes that are required by a growing body for many functions, mainly growth and repair of tissues, building stronger bones and joints, and even to prevent phlegm that is associated with cold, sinus, flu, etc. So the dal that you are forcing them to eat for protein has stuff that comes in the way of protein assimilation. The dal that you are forcing them to eat to become strong could even be making them sick frequently.

The reason why kids are happy to eat legumes like chana, rajma, sundals and usals is because these go through a process of soaking, fermentation and thorough cooking that helps remove these natural inhibitors, thus improving both taste and nutrient levels of the meal.

So really, all you need is regular home-cooked, wholesome meals, the same old local, seasonal, belonging to food heritage, and these more than meet a growing child's protein requirement.

The three pillars for protein synthesis and assimilation are a) frequent and timely meals (those recesses and meal breaks are there for a reason), b) activity and play (especially lost games that challenge the full body strength like kho-kho, langdi, even kandaphodi where you learn to jump over each other's bodies) and c) regulated, early bedtime.

You get these three in place, you get the protein, fuel their growth and keep them disease-free. The rest is just bakwas.

As for dal, if you really do want to feed it to them, pre-soak it for at least thirty minutes before cooking. This allows for the anti-nutrient levels to drop. Also, do know in your hearts, that even just rice and salt and ghee along with the three pillars will more than do the job. And as they get eight and older, they naturally return to eating dals, so for now, chill.

3. Vitamins from greens

i could barely control my nausea. My friend was feeding her eight-month-old salad greens at a trendy café in Bangalore. i could barely look at the poor child. 'i have taught him to eat everything,' she said proudly. i forced a smile but i wanted to strangle my friend.

If parents who say there's protein in dal tend to feel that their children eat nothing, then parents who say that spinach mein iron hai are also the ones who are busy making variety for dinner. Variety means anything that is not local, regional or traditional. So, they may whip up a pasta or tortilla or khow suey, and occasionally a pav bhaji and then add all kinds of vegetables to these things. Then to wash away their own guilt for not cooking regular food, they serve these things with a dose of healthy salad — often raw, unrecognisable veggies, mixed with each other in a big salad bowl.

The truth, though, is again the same: even if roti-ghee-jaggery, dahi-rice-achaar, khichdi-papad, poha, paratha, etc. are not taught or positioned as sources of vitamins and minerals, they very much are. Our ignorance about their goodness doesn't make the goodness vanish. It very much stays in there and in forms that can be easily assimilated.

Green leafy veggies and raw veggies have the same issue as dal — anti-nutrients that come in the way of vitamin and mineral absorption. Of course, a young body with strong survival instincts wants to optimise its chances for a good, healthy life and refuses to bite into the salad. But you still force, so the poor thing is down with regular allergies, infections, intolerances, etc. Cooking veggies the way they are meant to be cooked, using traditional recipes with tadkas of herbs, spices and even legumes (like peanuts, etc.), reduces the anti-nutrient value and makes the nutrients more available for absorption. So does following basic rules of the season like not eating green leafy vegetables during monsoon as the soil is not suitable for their growth at that point. Also, as children grow up to five years and beyond, teach them to try one teaspoon of everything that is cooked at home. That will allow them to expand their palate, not feel forced to eat quantities of sabzi and also ensure that diversity of the diet is maintained.

And if you are still hung up on vitamins and minerals — all traditional halwas, barfis and laddoos are full of them. In fact, they are better sources of these micronutrients than sabzis as they contain essential fat — either in the form of ghee or dry fruit — which allows for fat-soluble vitamins (A, E, D, K) to be absorbed and for the gut to get strong enough to assimilate the minerals. So yes, salads and soups are both unnecessary additions to the daily diet and only add to daily drama over food.

BROCCOLI IN MANALI

You do mota mota know that climate change is affecting the growth of many crops in regions across the globe. Closer to home, Manali or even Simla are no longer the largest producers of apples. The case is that much starker in Manali. With forests being cut to grow more apples (it's a cash crop), the temperatures in the region rose and with that the yield fell. Now the bigger producer is a region much higher than Manali — Keylong in Lahaul.

The other interesting thing is what is happening between the apple trees in Manali. So earlier, if they would grow all local veggies or even allow wild uncultivated species to crop up, the space is now completely taken over by 'angrezi sabzi' — broccoli and the likes. These are for the consumption of the elite of Delhi but pollute the pristine Manali. The soil, water and

> air are damaged by the chemical fertilisers and pesticide sprays needed to grow broccoli. And its people are denied their local sabzi or even millets like kodra, and what's worse, nobody in the metros is getting magically thin or healthier eating broccoli either.

Important note: Eating spicy food

First of all, a lot of us attach unnecessary prestige to eating bland food. The British invaded India for its spices, and the rest, as they say, is history. In the present, the UK is selling turmeric latte, the US is drinking fennel or cinnamon tea, and the EU is discovering the therapeutic properties of chillies. We, in the meanwhile, are making saada paratha, feeding our kids vegetable sticks, and hoping that they guzzle down beetroot or cauliflower soup.

Spices, especially the way they are used in Indian kitchens, bring out the real flavour in food, increase the therapeutic value of the meal, and even enhance the gut microbiota diversity. Health 101 would also mean using spices in your kitchen. The fresher, the better. Ideally, we should expect that our children grow up with the ability and sharp senses to tell one spice from another by just smelling it or with one bite of the food. That's what well-raised children are like.

As for them having to deal with too many spices at

a guest's place, just teach them how to deal with it. Too teekha? Mix some salt with it, it takes away the sting. Still teekha? Sprinkle some nimbu, and you are good to go. Too salty? Add lime and a pinch of sugar. Too sweet? Eat some sugar and then eat it. There are a hundred ways to deal with it, and it's your responsibility to teach them how to eat it or bring it to the exact metric that they prefer. Then it's an empowered child, or else you are just raising someone who is going to be dependent on others to make it exactly the way he / she prefers to eat it. Recipe for disaster, if you ask me. Besides, here's a life lesson Mamai taught me, it's gross but invaluable and teaches you how to behave when you are a guest — *aapla ghar hagun bhar, dusryacha ghar thuki la dar*. Shit all you want in your own house but when in other people's homes, behave properly, as even your spit will be taxed. Entitled and brattish behaviour is not cool and it's never too early to teach that.

There are a hundred different challenges that your child is going to face in the real world — spices or masala should really be the least of your concerns. And i already told you, if you want to raise a happy child, teach them the value of food. It takes a lot of effort to put food on the table; if one day there's too much of something in any dish, no big deal, take it in your stride. Especially when you are a guest, compliment the host for everything that they have cooked, and mean it. That's the recipe to happiness, and happy kids are healthy kids.

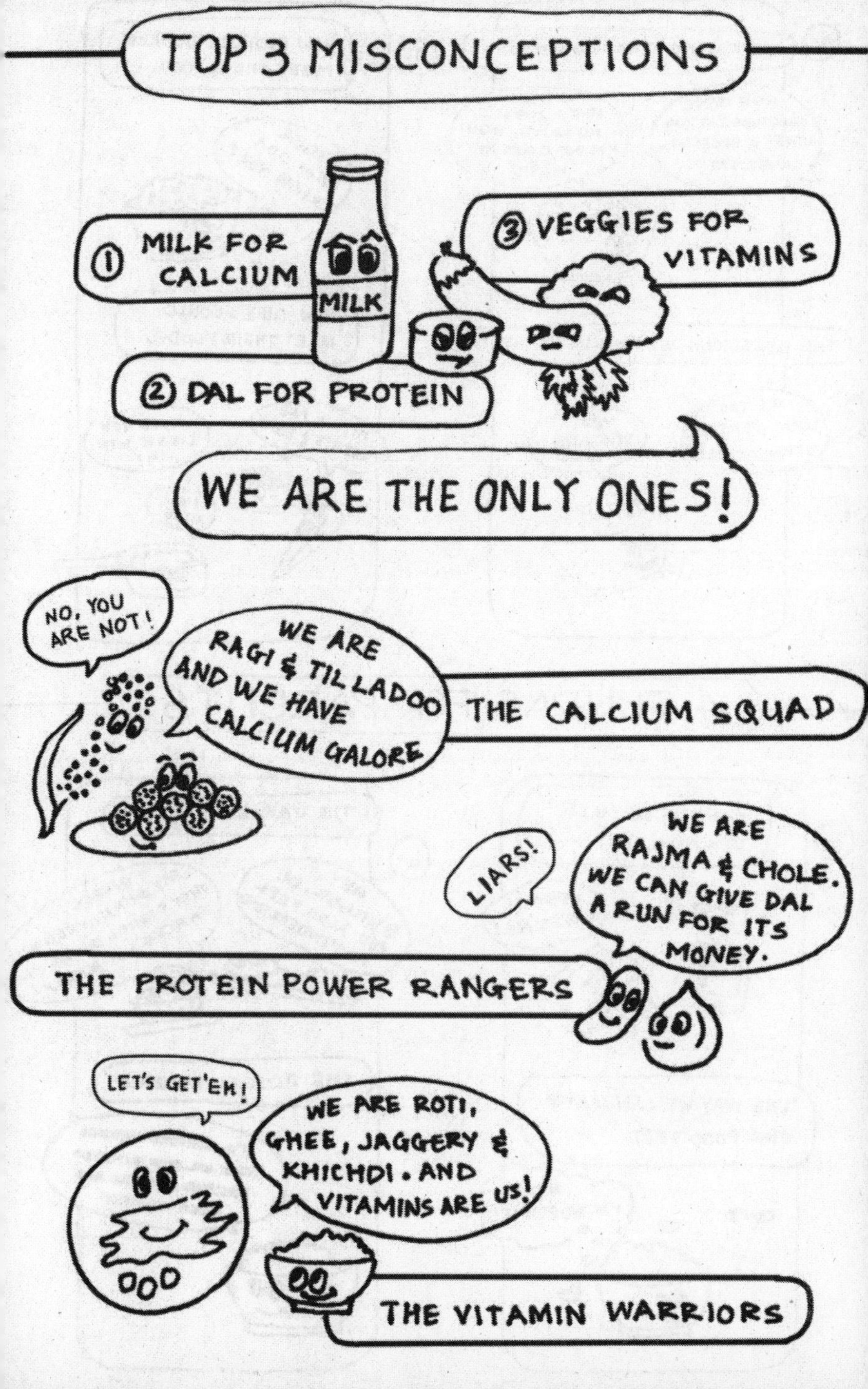
TOP 3 MISCONCEPTIONS
① MILK FOR CALCIUM
MILK
② DAL FOR PROTEIN
③ VEGGIES FOR VITAMINS
WE ARE THE ONLY ONES!
NO, YOU ARE NOT!
WE ARE RAGI & TIL LADOO AND WE HAVE CALCIUM GALORE
THE CALCIUM SQUAD
LIARS!
WE ARE RAJMA & CHOLE. WE CAN GIVE DAL A RUN FOR ITS MONEY.
THE PROTEIN POWER RANGERS
LET'S GET'EM!
WE ARE ROTI, GHEE, JAGGERY & KHICHDI. AND VITAMINS ARE US!
THE VITAMIN WARRIORS

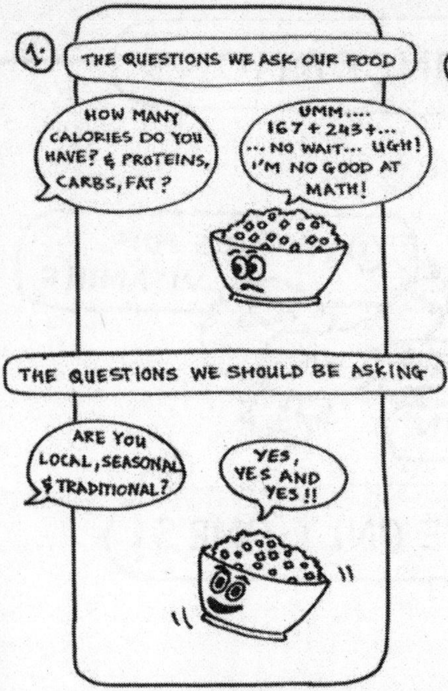
1.
THE QUESTIONS WE ASK OUR FOOD
HOW MANY CALORIES DO YOU HAVE? & PROTEINS, CARBS, FAT?
UMM.... 167 + 243 +... ... NO WAIT... UGH! I'M NO GOOD AT MATH!
THE QUESTIONS WE SHOULD BE ASKING
ARE YOU LOCAL, SEASONAL & TRADITIONAL?
YES, YES AND YES !!

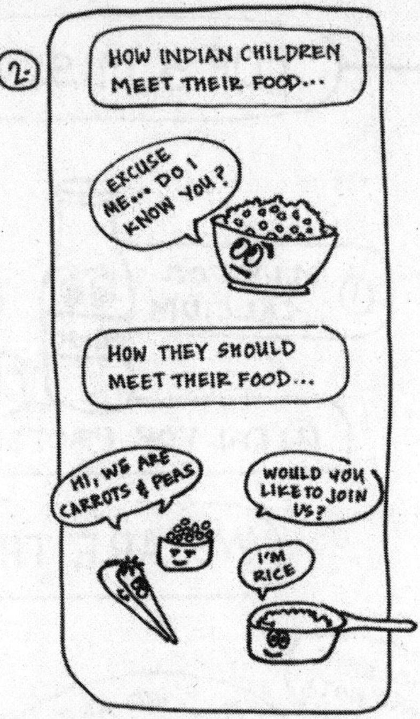
2.
HOW INDIAN CHILDREN MEET THEIR FOOD...
EXCUSE ME... DO I KNOW YOU?
HOW THEY SHOULD MEET THEIR FOOD...
HI, WE ARE CARROTS & PEAS
WOULD YOU LIKE TO JOIN US?
I'M RICE

4 FUNDAS FOR PARENTS

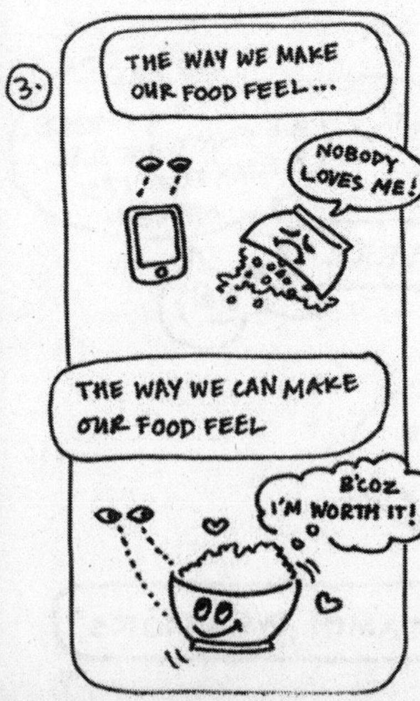
3.
THE WAY WE MAKE OUR FOOD FEEL...
NOBODY LOVES ME!
THE WAY WE CAN MAKE OUR FOOD FEEL
B'COZ I'M WORTH IT!

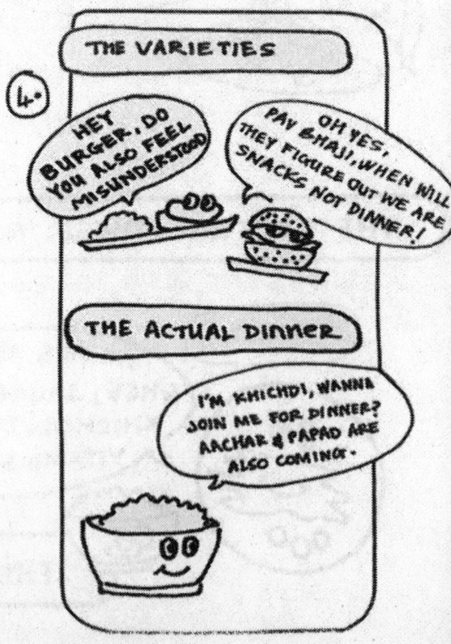
4.
THE VARIETIES
HEY BURGER, DO YOU ALSO FEEL MISUNDERSTOOD
OH YES, PAV BHAJI, WHEN WILL THEY FIGURE OUT WE ARE SNACKS NOT DINNER!
THE ACTUAL DINNER
I'M KHICHDI, WANNA JOIN ME FOR DINNER? AACHAR & PAPAD ARE ALSO COMING.

Chapter 2
For Kids — Making Right Food Decisions

On the New Year's Eve of 2015, i was in Naggar, a small village near Manali, with thirty, fourteen-year-old kids. They were part of my partner's New Year trip, during which they went skiing, trekking and mountain biking. i just joined them for a couple of days. Being a teenager is always tough, but in 2015 it seemed much tougher, and with time it's only getting more ruthless. You have adult bodies but childlike brains and even softer hearts.

There were five teachers as part of this group, and the school had a strict no cell phone on trips policy. The two nights that i was there, the teachers raided the kids' bags in the night and found four cell phones on one day and two on the next. The parents had insisted that the kids carry their phones despite the school's policy, and even though teachers sent regular updates on the WhatsApp parent groups about the well-being of the kids and the trip in general. 'Oh, come on,' one of the students protested, 'we are using the phone as a camera'; Sorry, that is also not allowed, was the reply. Phew! Never before had parents actively encouraged children to bypass school rules (even if it came out of concern for their safety, misplaced i think, very much), and never before had a phone also worked as a camera. 'Tough hai ya,' i said to GP. 'Teachers ke liye?' he asked (both his parents are government school teachers). 'Students ke liye,' i said, even though half my family are school teachers.

Then there's the food part. No junk food was allowed: the school has a no junk food policy and so does Connect with Himalaya, GP's venture. Khakra, thepla, the Gujju stuff was allowed, and we were in the Himalaya, so fresh food was easily available. But there were chips, chocolates, biscuits found during the phone raid. It's not that these kids were eager to eat unhealthy — they were amongst the brightest, most curious and enthusiastic group that i had ever interacted with. But they just didn't know better. Also, parenting these days has changed — the parents had packed the junk food for them lest they go hungry because they didn't like the food that was on offer. Unknowingly, we treat kids like consumers, always trying to make them happy, keep them entertained and, worse, seek their approval. A teenager's brain is still developing, so they respond by manipulating the parents in return, and lo and behold, you have a disaster.

The kids complained that there wasn't enough snow to ski, drank only mineral water, even when the hotel provided clean drinking water, and found the local food too spicy (Himachali food isn't spicy but flavourful). Then, on my second night there, even without wanting to say anything, the kids received a full thirty-minute lecture from me at dinner. The setting was beautiful. We were in the dining room of the ancient Naggar castle, nestled between snow-covered peaks, the wide open valley and the Beas river below us, and all that the garam khun wanted was pizza or noodles or at least pav bhaji. Irony was smiling upon us. i said many things to them, but mostly i told them about:

- How rich kids are the problem. How impoverished must we be to come to a beautiful setting like this, and complain about how the snow is not enough.
- About how chocolates were a poor way to fill one's stomach and are not a replacement for dinner; and how chocolate companies employ poor children from poor countries, denying them a shot at childhood.
- About how when the girls in the group were having black coffee without sugar instead of eating breakfast in the hope of losing weight, all i felt was pity, because they must have the confidence to allow their bodies to grow and ditch boys or girl friends who find them fat.
- About ketchup and how it has the least amount of nutrients and masks the taste of all flavours, leaving

us unable to enjoy Himalayan flavours or food.

- About how, at fourteen, they should be able to think about where this plastic bottle goes after they leave from here. Does the country or even the world have the capacity to recycle?
- About how water and cola companies have depleted the water resources of the earth, especially in developing countries, and how it took three to seven litres from common public resources to make one litre of a cola, and how this is an ecological theft.

Blah, blah, blah, i ranted, and the kids listened in pin-drop silence. Just then, a man, unwitting witness to this whole food drama, sitting there with his two young boys — both under ten — and wife, stood up and clapped. i looked in his direction and said, 'Thank you, sir.' Post that, the kids and our entire group ate everything that was on offer.

The next morning, one of the teachers came up to me and said, 'Bohot accha kiya madam. We tell them all the time, but if someone from outside says they listen.' The mineral water didn't get bought the next day. One of the boys came up to me and said, 'Ma'am, it's not that we don't understand and it won't be immediate, but we will give up on chocolates.' Oh! My heart melted; i could have cried, i could have danced with joy, but since i am a Konkanastha, i nodded my head and said, 'Yes, i know.' Anybody who says that teenagers are heartless or clueless just hasn't spent time with them.

Identifying unhealthy food

So, anyway, in the absence of parental guidance or more like in the presence of confusion, schools dishing out lopsided views on what is healthy and food companies promising to send us to Paris for buying their biscuits, colas or cereals, how do we decide what is good for us? It's actually not all that hard once you begin to tell the patterns. You have all watched enough crime dramas or read enough suspense thrillers to tell what the plot actually is, na? So here goes first: what to not buy, what to not eat and what is not a gift or a treat:

1. Does it come in a packet that is available across the globe or pan India? Mass produced.
2. Does the packaging have a diagram of any body part — brain, bicep or shows a growing body? Grabs attention and plays on your vulnerabilities — you are not smart or strong or tall enough.
3. Does it claim to be rich in a nutrient or have extra doses of a nutrient? Iron, fibre, protein, vitamin D? Textbook nutritionism (read previous chapter or ask your parents about it once they have read it).
4. Is it giving you a free toy for buying the product or a chance to win an iPhone or an all-expenses paid foreign trip? Illegal in a lot of countries where governments are active in protecting children from the cheap and unethical marketing practices of food companies.
5. Does your favourite movie star or cricketer endorse

the product? Truth be told, you are only engaged as a brand ambassador of junk food when you have a fit and agile body. Essentially, it means that you have had the mental and physical discipline to stay away from the very food that you are endorsing. And to tell you a secret, the celebs won't even consume it on the day of the shoot; they only act like they slurped, drank or ate, never even once letting it down their throats. Call it occupational hazard, if you must.

So any 'food' that meets even three of the above criteria fits the pattern of profits over people. It is poor for your health, poor for the economy (doesn't support local businesses) and poor for our global ecology (leaves behind a carbon footprint and makes unaccountable use of natural resources).

Almost all juices, cereals, colas, biscuits (even the fibre-rich ones), chips (yeah, even the multi-grain, baked ones), chocolates, etc., fall in this category. So do burgers, pizzas, ice creams and even sandwiches or salad companies that operate across the globe. It is invariably these businesses that also make the most noise about generating employment or providing free education to the poor in your country. The word for this is deflection; they are simply distracting you from what they are really doing — making profits at the cost of your health, at the cost of local businesses or economy and at the cost of global ecology: our collective resources of forests, fresh water and fertile land.

CELEB ENDORSEMENTS AND SOCIAL MEDIA INFLUENCERS

You've got to realise that some people in some professions — cricket, acting, etc., are going to have a bigger share of limelight and fame than most others. That doesn't mean that the people working in these industries are not sensitive or sensible human beings. Virat Kohli refused to extend his contract with Pepsico — that should have earned him adulation, front page headlines and full page editorials. Instead it got treated like a Harris shield score in newspapers.

Basically, going after celebs for junk food endorsements is like screaming at the telemarketing executive because they put you on hold for twenty minutes. It may make you feel good for five minutes, or in the case of celebs, have the topic trend for two days at the most, but then it's business as usual. You need to take the same approach that you take with the telemarketing executive: 'How do i escalate my complaint?' Take the exact same approach with celeb endorsements; they may make millions but are the lowest common denominator in this game. Government, junk food industry, policies — we should be barking up that tree. As for celebs, they love popularity (we all do, actually), so once there is momentum in public opinion, they will stay away from junk food ads.

Then there is the ever-evolving game of social media posts, trends and retweets. On the one hand, it has opened a new career as a social media influencer; on the other, the lines between genuine advice and paid promotions are invisible. Almost everything that you see, from magazine covers, photo shoots, candid posts to even campaigns like #beyourself or whatever, all have an agenda of selling / monetising at the cost of the naïve follower. The least you should expect from anyone you follow online is that they make it clear if a recommendation is genuine or paid. You can then make an informed decision as you deem fit.

Identifying what to eat: The three tests

So then what is the food that you can eat? Well, that's a simpler one to answer, and these three tests will help you make the right food choices.

1. *Does it pass the grandmom test?* It has two parts: a) Does your grandmom recognise this item as food? b) Did your grandmom eat this when she was your age?

Oats, your grandmom may recognise now, she may also recognise pasta, or even a brownie or a doughnut as food, but she never had it when she was your age. And she may not have even known of its existence till you came along and there's a good chance that though she may have bought this for you, she's never even tasted it and has no intentions of doing so in the future. So yup, talk to your grandmom, and if you don't have one, talk to anyone of your grandmom's age. A friend's dadi / nani, someone you sat next to on a flight or ask in school to arrange a grandmom or granddad day for a freewheeling chat on food.

2. *Does it have a local name?* If yes, this ensures that the food that you are eating is a native of the land that you are living in. That it has adapted to its climate, has the nutrients that you need to fuel your growth (and prevent diseases), is ecologically smart because it has not travelled a long distance to land on your plate. So, other than being good for your health, it is also good for your farmer or local economy.

Now this will help you catch anything that is of value to you, but may be out of your radar or that of your parents' because it doesn't get written about or has still not been discovered by the West and paraded around like the answer to all your problems. Gond and aliv laddoo, rajgeera chiki, kodra roti, samo chawal, kokum sherbet, amla moramba are just some of the things that quickly come to one's mind.

On the other hand, it also allows you to see through

a lot of exotic foods that have no health, economical or ecological value to you. E.g. quinoa, cranberries, kiwi, kale, soya beans, broccoli, rucola, etc. Local language mein kya bolta hai? That's an important question that you must ask and get an answer to. And real gold is the food that only has a local name but no angrezi equivalent; that's the stuff the UNFAO calls NUS — neglected and underutilised species. Food stuff that is great but currently not valued in its region or country of origin because of poor prestige or lack of information associated with it. Most of this stuff belongs to developing regions, like Asia, Africa, Latin America. And then it invariably gets taken to the richer regions, introduced as novel food, and then the whole world can't wait to copy it. More details in my book *Indian Super Foods*, but quick examples are turmeric latte (India), quinoa (Latin America), Rooibos tea (Africa).

3. *Does it have multiple uses / is versatile?* The healthiest food is that which can be used in a variety of manners; its versatility is its strength. It's like the playground in school: you can use it to run on, to conduct annual days on, to host a festival or exhibition. Or like your granddad: you can eat with him, chill with him, travel with him, etc. If people or food are uni-dimensional, it is the biggest giveaway; it tells you that they are not so great after all. Being an all-rounder is important. Food that can be used in a variety of ways is the real definition of super food. Everything else is just food business.

MY OXFORD KID

Everything that i know about economics, both macro or micro, is because of one of my young clients who studies in Oxford. Her whole class comprises super-intelligent, driven people with the craft to look at numbers with one eye on creativity and another on reality. Just her diet recall made for wonderful reading; her ability to interpret her own data, predict what that would mean for the next day, next week or period cycle, left me in awe. She surely taught me a thing or two, but the best thing that she told me was about her roommates, two Italian boys. 'Lucky girl,' i teased her, 'lots of pizza and pasta coming your way.' 'Ah, no!' she said. 'They won't make it because the water, pasta and seasonings, i.e., ingredients (or data), are not up to the mark.' So they helped her make aloo gobhi, took turns making rajma-rice, but pizza and pasta were kept for Italy. Shabbash, i wholeheartedly endorse and approve of this intelligent behaviour, of not making compromises with life's essentials. Sher bukha marega but ghaas nahi khayega; well raised boys, i tell you. Oxford, you lucky thing, you. Aur hum log? Idhar pasta and Italy mein khakra ;-).

Let's look at a few examples:

Banana — the stalk and raw banana can be turned into a sabzi, the ripe one is eaten as a fruit or turned into a milkshake, the overripe one is turned into a sheera or halwa. The leaf is used as a plate (ecologically smart) and brings easy money for the farmer (economically sensitive to sections in need of help), the branch is used as a mandap for poojas.

Mango — raw for achaar, ripe as fruit or aamras, overripe for aam paapad or golis, leaves for decoration or poojas, bark for its medicinal purposes, wood for lightweight furniture.

Rice — kheer, rice, pulao, biryani, atta for rotis or dosa, base for idlis, modak. Uncooked rice in rituals, rice husk and hay for cattle feed, rice paste for rangoli, dried rice still in the hay as door décor.

Milk — plain, kharwas, dahi, chaas, lassi, sheera, kheer, solvent for therapeutic ingredients like dried ginger powder, haldi, etc.

Ber – ripe eaten as a fruit or with some kalanamak as a snack, tree used as a fence.

Basically, food that is good for you:

- Should be eaten in more ways than one
- Should have a ritualistic or decorative purpose
- Should have a therapeutic or medicinal value

When most of the food you eat through the day has all three or at least two applications in the day-to-day life of your region, then what you are eating is super healthy.

Four food habits of healthy kids

Alright, so based on everything that we have discussed above, here are four practical steps to ensure that you stay strong, smart and sensible with food. i am calling them four food habits of healthy kids:

1. Nothing out of a packet for breakfast

This means no packaged cereals (including oats), no juices, breads, noodles, etc. Not only are they low on nutrition, they are, in fact, harmful for your health. The low quality–high quantity sugar (mostly HFCS or corn syrup), chemical preservatives, emulsifiers, etc., hamper the growth of your body and mind. They also don't pass any of the tests mentioned above.

So what can you eat? Oh, there are so many good options — tasty and healthy; one of the benefits of living in an ancient and evolved food culture like ours. Poha, upma, idli, dosa, wada, thepla, khakra, paratha, jolpan, siddu, missi roti, and many more from the treasure trove of diverse Indian breakfasts with their even more diverse accompaniments. They are prepared fresh, eaten hot and are in tune with the season and even genetically compliant. They fuel you in the right way for the long hours of school ahead and don't drain you or make you dull like packaged foods will invariably do. As they say, well begun is half done.

If you go to school early and don't feel like or have time for a full breakfast, a glass of milk (not Tetra Pak) or a fresh fruit along with a handful of dry fruits will also do. More details in Part 2.

DESIGNER FOOD MOLECULES AND GRAS

Chemistry is a beautiful thing and food chemistry even more so. While there are many applications of food chemistry, one of the most controversial applications has been to create what is called as designer food molecules. These molecules don't exist in nature but are created in labs to add, retain or enhance the flavour of food. They are also used to add texture and freshness to food; essentially, artificially enhance the taste experience of ultra-processed packaged food. Ever wondered why when a fresh fruit is cut open, it will decay and perish within hours, but fruit juice packets that last almost forever continue to call themselves 'free of preservatives'? Well, it's the designer food molecules at work. And you are probably the first generation that is consuming them with regularity and intensity. It will take a long time to figure the exact extent of the damage that it has done to your system and the food industry will fight tooth and nail to blame everything other than their products for this damage. But that doesn't take away from the fact that from tooth decay to kidney stones, fatty liver to high triglycerides, obesity to diabetes, we are seeing it all in kids as young as six.

Take anything that you really like and read the package contents, the small print, from infant baby formulas to ketchup, from juices to colas, from caffeinated energy drinks to biscuits, from chocolate-coated cereals to almond milk, you will see ingredients that are identified as an alphabet followed by a number and some chemical names that clearly don't sound like food. That's the designer food molecules, buddies, and countries like the mighty US have a way of legalising them and allowing them in the human food chain; it's called GRAS — generally regarded as safe.

This GRAS certificate is not earned through an independent, non-biased food certification agency, but is given by the food company to itself (it's like giving yourself a good conduct certificate). It's just some paperwork, and then stuff that has no history of being consumed as food by mankind finds its way on your table and finally into your tiny stomach.

P.S.: Stevia is GRAS.

Can you think of five breakfast ideas that meet the grandmom test, local name and versatility rules, and which support your health, economy and ecology?

2. No plastic dabbas or bottles in schools

Now, of course, our wannabe giri doesn't just stop at adopting the cheap cereal-and-packaged milk or packaged juices over the priceless diverse array of Indian breakfasts and meals. It extends itself to cheap cutlery too, right from the infant stage. Walk into any 5-star, and you will find an awkward-looking maid feeding a little baby from a garish plastic dabba and spoon. First of all, once you grow up and even now, speak up for the rights of all those who are unable to speak for themselves, especially within your home, school and society. And secondly, know that plastic is not a great material — it may have some very unique applications in some areas of life, but with food, none whatsoever.

And we don't just stop at plastic dabbas and bottles, we even have cling film that chipkaos to the food we eat, and aluminium foil that wraps itself around rotis and sandwiches. Basically, we do really cheap things to appear rich or even neat. In the process, we impoverish our diverse microbiome ecosystem (gut-friendly bacteria) and immune response, and contaminate our bodies with toxic agents like the xenoestrogens (chemical compounds similar to the estrogen hormone which confuse the body) in plastic which leach into your food. Together with aluminium that interferes with the absorption of important minerals like zinc, plastic blunts our testosterone, growth hormones and insulin response. All in all, we start looking rounder and get weaker instead of leaner and stronger as we grow. Our hormones are all messed up even before they have had the chance to strike that right balance.

So what can you use?

In all ancient cultures, when the baby turns around six months old and goes from an exclusive diet of mother's milk to also eating what mother nature has to offer, there is a ceremony. Typically, in this ceremony, depending on the region you come from, your mama or nani or another designated close relative gifts the baby silverware. Usually a small plate, bowl and a glass. This time-honoured tradition is not just an occasion to celebrate the baby reaching a milestone, but also to ensure protection from viral and bacterial infections, as silver has been used to fight infections long before antibiotics were discovered.

Of course, silver is a one-time, expensive investment,

but it does prove itself to be economical in the long run, as it leads to: a) building an asset (precious metals typically appreciate in value) b) building memories, as the silverware will invariably have the family name carved on it, and maybe even a unique design to boot c) prevent illnesses and protection against use of antibiotics (you all know their ill effects, right? Especially related to loss of friendly gut bacteria). Incidentally, this is also the age when diversity of friendly bacteria starts building up.

Eating fresh, seasonal and regional food in non-toxic material like silver, kansa or even steel and glass, helps in building and nurturing a diverse gut bacteria ecosystem. Loss of diversity in the microbiota, especially in little kids, is also positively associated with incidences of Type 1 diabetes, autism, asthma, obesity, slower brain and cognitive development and language skills — the list is endless.

3. *No gadgets while eating*

All human beings are born with the ability to self-terminate the act of eating. Not just humans, all animals and birds, all living beings, in fact, instinctively know how much to eat at a time. When you were an infant, no matter what, you would not drink a drop of milk more than you needed. Even when you started having solid food, it was really tough for your parents to overfeed you as you would throw up anything extra. So why, then, by the time you became an adolescent, and later an adult, did how much food to eat and where to stop become a big task or something that someone else, a dietitian for example, has to tell you? Because we are now distracted when we eat and no longer listen to the signals from the stomach. Deep down, in the gut, in the stomach, there's a brain, sharper and braver than the one in your head, and it speaks to you when you are silent. So tune in and practise listening when you are eating, that's when it speaks the loudest. If you are on a gadget — whether it's the phone, iPad or TV — all that you do is end up consuming much more than you need. And now you already know food can also consume you, so stay careful with that relationship and don't let it turn toxic.

TV DINNERS

As the income of an Indian family increases, their consumption patterns change — of everything, including food. It's not uncommon these days to find homes with more than one TV, and the largest screen is positioned strategically across the dining table in the living room. This is where families proudly tell you that they eat together, but scratch the surface, they only consume some food along with a lot of propaganda on news or some shaitan, nagin TV serial together. All families now have TV sets in bedrooms too, but some families take it a notch higher and even sprawl on the bed in the reclining Vishnu posture with their plates kept on old newspaper (bed saaf rakhne ke liye) so they can eat while watching TV. There should be an award for maintaining the anantasana while watching TV and eating at the same time, but there is none, unless you would like to count obesity as one of your achievements. And if you are richer than the middle class, there is a high chair and a personal iPad or iPhone, who knows even Apple TV, for the kid.

The point is, it's not about where you are sitting — on a high chair, at the dining table or sprawling across the bed. If you are viewing something while eating, you have already dug yourself a hole from which health cannot bloom. When it's food, it should be just you and the food, a real conversation with a real person at most, not on FaceTime or WhatsApp video.

There's a hormone called leptin that gets released once the stomach is full. If you are distracted, you will not notice or pay attention to the signal of leptin. And then, instead of stopping at the right place, you will either overeat or under-eat, or eat just to get some dominating adult who has made stuffing you the main aim of their life off your back.

Let them get a life and, in the meanwhile, you focus all your senses on eating. In my view, this is meditation for children — eating with all our senses.

And if your mommy or anybody tells you that for finishing everything on your plate you will get fifteen minutes of extra TV, hold one hand over your heart and vigorously shake the other by holding it in front of your face and say, 'No, no dear, don't be so cheap. Gadget is not a gift.'

4. No chocolates or ice creams post dinner

This should be simple enough, but it's not quite. First of all, you do know that post sunset digestion slows down, and this isn't exactly the time to load your system with some mass-produced, industrialised product, be it chocolate, ice cream or even that store-bought cupcake. Take a break, and do a quick reality check. Do you even love what you are eating or are you eating it because it's a cool thing to do, comes with a toy or the face of your favourite cartoon character, or is endorsed by a celeb you love? i mean, figure out — is this actual love for what you are eating or is this manipulation by the food industry? Or are you being manipulated by your parent? Is it a treat to finish everything on your plate or a compensation for not making your favourite sabzi or some other kind of trade-off? Because if it is, your parent is just being weak. Firstly, you should know that appetite changes every day and you don't have to finish everything that's laid out. Secondly, it's ok, sometimes a favourite thing is cooked, sometimes not; you don't have to be compensated for the natural workings of the kitchen and then be called a spoilt brat behind your back. You get the drift?

You don't need me to say this, but there really is nothing healthy about a cola, ice cream, chocolate post a meal, especially post dinner. You land up having them either because someone has preyed on your childlike judgement, or because it's a part of the meal deal, like it's free with a pizza or burger. Dinner is the last meal before sleep, and good quality of sleep is critical to all parameters of growth — emotional, intellectual and physical; you don't want to mess with that. So ensure that dinners are meals that help you get into a steady state — both mentally and physically. It must have a repetitive value, something like dal-chawal or khichdi or roti-sabzi type: wholesome, flavoured and spiced just right. So that it allows for a good quality of the other repetitive, critical act of uninterrupted, undisturbed sleep.

Your need to have these stimulants is also the highest when you are fed a steady diet of variety for dinner — aaj pav bhaji, kal pasta, parso Chinese. So, also spend some time figuring out what are the triggers for wanting these stimulants, and you will discover that post a meal of khichdi or just dal-rice-ghee or a roti / bhakri-sabzi and chaas, you feel at your lightest and most content, and least interested in a chocolate, ice cream, etc. The key, of course, is to observe yourself, and for that, the gadget should be switched off, as we have already learnt.

Stimulants are best limited to once a month or even less, and have them before 6 p.m. so that they don't come in the way of your sleep. Same thing with variety — finish before 6 p.m. so that the excesses of just one kind of taste in that meal don't keep you awake with thirst or gastric disturbances in the night. And always eat these meals in a way that allows you to have your repetitive and valuable dinner and sleep on time.

If you are hungry post dinner, a glass of milk with freshly powdered nuts, kesar and sugar or jaggery is a great meal, which allows you to have something sweet but doesn't stimulate you or disturb the natural hormonal cycle and leave you with disturbed sleep.

THE HIERARCHY OF SWEETS

As far as homemade halwas, laddoos and barfis go, know that they don't even qualify as desserts and therefore don't have the same bad news around them: disturbed sleep or obesity and unstable blood sugars. The grains or the millets in them, along with the pulses, nuts, ghee, seeds, spices and sugar or jaggery, make for a nutrient-dense meal. A smart marketing brain would have called it energy balls or ancient bars or power powders (for halwas), but we have regional names for them, and in the age of marketing, these don't seem to be cool enough, even though they very much are. So you can have these as a mid-day meal at school, or right after sports or even for breakfast, like laddoo and milk.

The stuff that you buy from local mithai shops — rasgullas, gulab jamuns, shrikhand (these are always better made at home though) — can be had occasionally, and even as a part of lunch or right after lunch. Do patronise the local halwai; these small businesses are fast losing ground to the cupcake churners that are taking out every corner shop out there. Trust me, just ten years ago, no one knew what a cupcake even was, or what the profession of a baker meant. But now it's some high-profile career and being a halwai is not. A halwai needs as much if not much more skill than a baker, but then he is not English-speaking, doesn't have an Instagram account or take pictures of his stuff as he makes them. So we see him in a poor light, even though what he makes is not something generic and available across the globe, but is specific to just our region or city. And the cupcake or chocolate people, who could be making the same stuff that is available across the globe and maybe in much better quality than what they are offering, come across as real cool. Scratch the surface and check: are you falling for positioning or content? When i asked myself that question as a kid, i realised that i really was just falling for positioning and marketing, and ice cream and chocolates didn't really make my stomach dance in joy. And once i figured that, i divorced them. Inspired?

Anyway, here's the hierarchy of sweets in descending order of goodness:

i. Made at home — laddoo, barfi, chiki, halwa, sheera, etc. — ok for all meals and for snacks too. Also post exercise.

ii. Same stuff as above, but made in a small co-operative or a family-run business — it's close enough to homemade. Don't have for breakfast though; that still needs to be something made in your kitchen only.

iii. India-specific mithai from local shops — occasionally, with lunch or as a mid-day meal.

Don't eat these for more than two to three days at a go. Most likely to happen during a festival like Diwali or some celebration like a shaadi. So when you buy, share with all, and keep only that much that won't last you for more than two, max three days. Post that, stop, even if you still have some at home. This much is already enough. i would also put local, small bakeries that make nankatais, mawa cakes, tuti-frutis in this category.

iv. Small shops or chefs that make cupcakes, cookies, chocolates, etc. (the Indian mithais, but made by large producers and available pan India and across select malls across the globe will also come in this category). You can have these cupcakes and cookies if they are served at your friend's birthday or a small piece occasionally, but only before 6 p.m., please. Know that these are not nutrient-rich enough for a growing body, even in their 'healthy' version. But definitely don't have them for festivals — celebrate with the sweets that your grandma did. They will have season-specific benefits; besides, these are rare, just in your part of the world, just your community, family: real gold.

v. Chocolates and ice creams — mass produced, available pan India and across the globe. This is the one that is the lowest in the hierarchy, along with colas and caffeinated energy drinks. Ideally, never touch at all. And if you must, rarely and always before 6 p.m. i won't spend much time talking about these, you already know it all by now. And hello, if you are a 5-star hotel manager and reading this and operating in India, please stop dishing out chocolates to our kids and make some richer, more priceless stuff instead. Can your chef whip up a nice, flavourful, marinated with nuts or coconut, halwa or a laddoo that only he or she can make and no one else can?

Important note: The hygiene hypothesis

The antibacterial soaps and the hand sanitisers may all be killing the bad bacteria (best case scenario) but are more likely to be making the pathogens or bad bacteria resistant to them, and with it killing all the good bacteria and messing up our hormonal environment / balance (real case scenario). The highly sanitised countries — US, UK, Australia, Singapore — have children with very high and sometimes even fatal levels of allergies. In the US, you are not allowed to take peanuts to school, and almost every café — even the smallest one selling muffins at a dingy corner at the airport — will declare that their products may contain allergens so you watch out for yourself.

Their paediatric associations are working hard to figure what's going wrong with the kids, and one of the reasons they have identified for these allergies, flus and infections is 'hygiene hypothesis'. Apart from being on packaged, processed diets, the kids live in such a sterilised environment that they have lost the diversity of the gut microbiota. This starts developing from an age as young as four to six months old. i heard a UK doctor speak at a conference, and he said that if we must build strong, resilient Brit kids, then we must let them be African in habits. What he meant was that we must allow our little kids to be picked up by aunts, uncles, neighbours; we must let them pick up the piece of fruit that fell on the floor and eat it; we must encourage them to go into muddy parks and roll around. And he said that he would even go to the extent of saying that we must let them gulp their own snort, at least once in a while. For us, this means letting Indian kids be more Indian. 'Look at this,' he pointed at the projector. The African kids had tiny little dots in all colours inside their stomachs and the Brit kids had a cluster of dots in just two colours in one corner. 'This, this lack of diverse bacteria, is costing our kids their childhood.' The US, btw, banned antibacterial soaps way back in September 2016. But then, from soaps to medicines, shampoos to toothpastes, a lot of stuff that is banned in other countries is dumped in ours, and legally at that. (You must have noticed the recent campaigns by these multinationals to 'improve' sanitation and health in our country.)

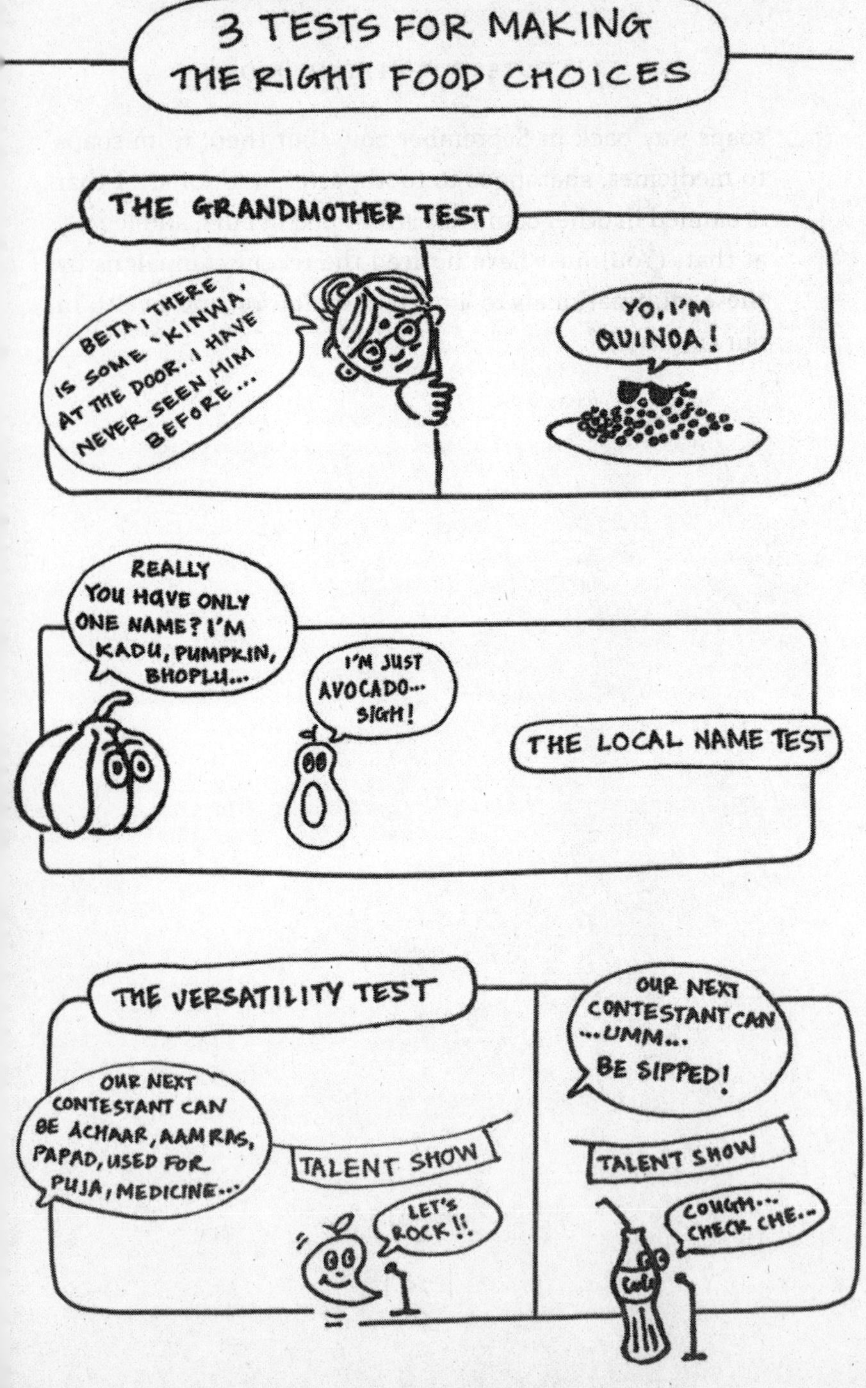
3 TESTS FOR MAKING THE RIGHT FOOD CHOICES
THE GRANDMOTHER TEST
BETA, THERE IS SOME 'KINWA' AT THE DOOR. I HAVE NEVER SEEN HIM BEFORE...
YO, I'M QUINOA!
REALLY YOU HAVE ONLY ONE NAME? I'M KADU, PUMPKIN, BHOPLU...
I'M JUST AVOCADO... SIGH!
THE LOCAL NAME TEST
THE VERSATILITY TEST
OUR NEXT CONTESTANT CAN BE ACHAAR, AAM RAS, PAPAD, USED FOR PUJA, MEDICINE...
TALENT SHOW
LET'S ROCK!!
OUR NEXT CONTESTANT CAN ...UMM... BE SIPPED!
TALENT SHOW
COUGH... CHECK CHE...

4 FOOD HABITS OF HEALTHY KIDS

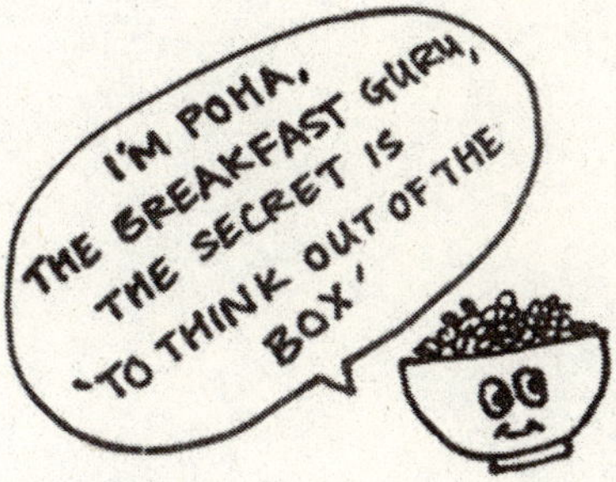
I'M POHA, THE BREAKFAST GURU, THE SECRET IS 'TO THINK OUT OF THE BOX.'

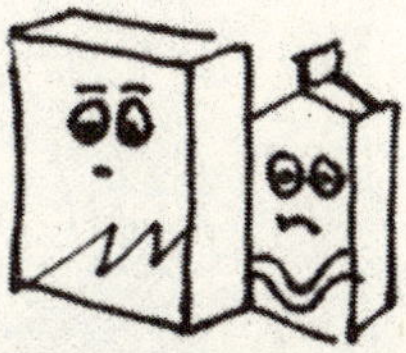

1. NOTHING OUT OF A PACKET FOR BREAKFAST

2. NO PLASTIC DABBAS OR BOTTLES IN SCHOOL.

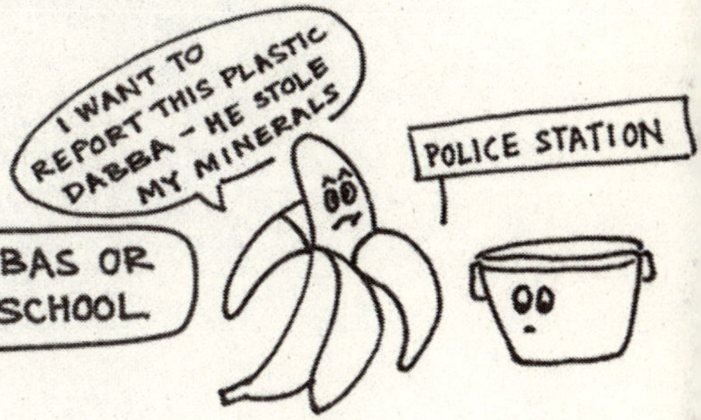
I WANT TO REPORT THIS PLASTIC DABBA - HE STOLE MY MINERALS
POLICE STATION

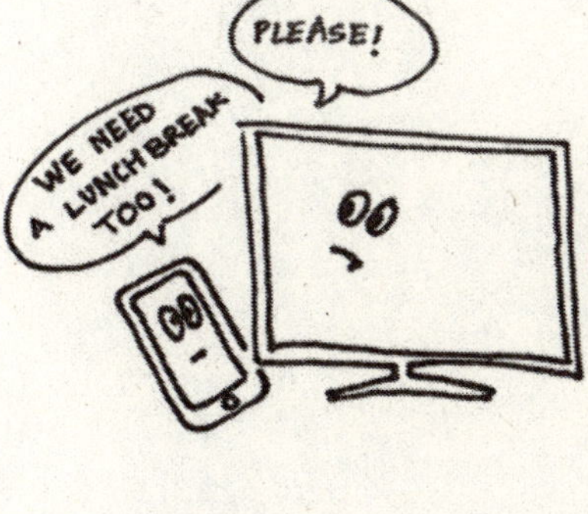
PLEASE!
WE NEED A LUNCH BREAK TOO!

3. NO GADGETS WHILE EATING

4. NO CHOCOLATES OR ICECREAMS POST DINNER

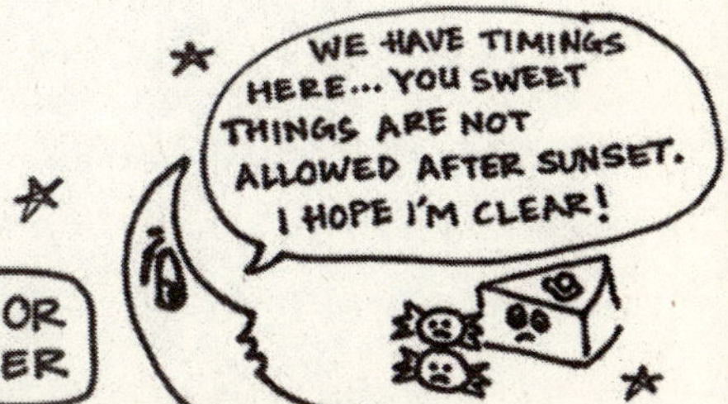
WE HAVE TIMINGS HERE... YOU SWEET THINGS ARE NOT ALLOWED AFTER SUNSET. I HOPE I'M CLEAR!

PART 1b: EXERCISE

Chapter 3

For Parents — Lead by Example

i was a part of a group of fourteen, trekking to the Changabang base camp in the Garhwal Himalaya. Not much is known about that area, and the first day ended up being too short a walk: we were at the campsite well before noon and had a lot of time to kill. The boys in the group decided that the little flat patch we had camped at was perfect to play cricket on. This is my worst time in mixed groups: when guys decide to have a ball and then the girls sit in one corner and chat, pretend to watch and have a good time. It puts me in an angry zone: i feel boys should know better and have the instinct of inclusion, but patriarchy buffers them from even the slightest sensitivity ... well, you don't want to know my trail of thoughts.

So, there were three women from Chennai, all in their forties, who were part of our group. One of them, Sheila, joined the boys and stood behind the wickets. Jhanvi, the enthu Gujju, joined too, fielding somewhere. i sat at a distance, crouched down, hating the world, the game of cricket and men at large. Just then, Sheila dived for the ball on her left, did a 180-degree somersault and flung the ball up in the air to celebrate the catch. 'Kaun hai re tu,' i said aloud as i clapped and walked towards her. 'What,' she asked, bewildered. 'Who are you,' i said more gently this time, gathering myself. 'Ah! That's Sheila Verghis, former cricketer,' shouted one of her friends, sipping chai. 'She stopped playing cricket ten years ago.' Shit, the game had changed for me. Once there's an athlete, a real one, someone who's cried in pain and joy over a game, i can watch and endlessly at that.

But other than the pure joy that it provides the spectator, what it gives the athlete is immeasurable. Sport is one thing that comes closest to spirituality, in more ways than one — it sets you free from the limitations of your body, of your gender, of biases, of prejudices, of everything that stops you from glory. And the thing is, irrespective of the money, glamour or visibility that it brings you, sports, any sport, sets you free.

i mean, what are most of us trying to do while earning money? Mostly we are trying to buy freedom, in the hope that it brings us the power to overcome all that limits us. i suspect that's what rich people are trying to do when they buy sports teams. But that's not how it works. Freedom from limitations is only earned through sweat, discipline and practice of the same stuff, over and over. So the twelfth man in a team is going to feel richer or more a part of the game than the team owner, even if it is the team owner's face that is regularly flashed across the screen.

Anyway, this is not about sports but about athleticism, which you can earn with free play also. Your child may never become a super athlete, but the fact that she has played a sport or a game (especially the unrecognised ones — lock and key, chor-police, langdi, etc.) will be useful for her years later.

WHY SHOULD YOUR CHILD PLAY / EXERCISE?

Raising healthy kids or parenting as an opportunity means ensuring that children have sixty to ninety minutes of free play every single day. There are immense benefits to this, and i am listing just a few.

Exercise / play/ sports:

1. Promotes the growth of butyrate-producing bacteria (friendly gut bacteria) that is critical for growth, hormones, immunity, etc.
2. Helps improve math scores and language skills (due to positive effects on learning centres in the brain).
3. Teaches the body to absorb and assimilate protein and calcium from food; makes digestion stronger.

4. Builds better neural pathways in the body and neurogenesis in the brain.
5. Builds stronger bones, tendons, ligaments — less chance of breaking anything when they fall.
6. Promotes accelerated recovery from all illnesses and traumas, be it mental or physical.
7. Prevents depression and channelises aggression (critical during the teenage years).
8. Keeps kids off toxic habits — drugs, alcohol, cigarettes, etc.
9. Teaches fair play, team work and respect for rules.
10. Keeps kids younger, innocent and childlike.
11. Teaches kids that losses and wins are impermanent and equips them with the ability to get over themselves.
12. Instils pride, self-esteem and self-discipline.

i could go on but will stop so that i can say there are literally a dozen reasons why your child should play every single day of her life. But, in real life, there are a dozen things that come in our way, especially if you live in cities and towns of India. In Sonave, my ancestral tribal village, the whole world is a playground. The kids may not have chappals on their feet, but they have mountains to climb, fields to run on and ponds to swim in. And all this within a safe environment and with the security of living within a community where everyone looks out for each other.

This is the model that we need to adopt in cities; we need to live better as communities (and we used to, until recently), so that one maid doesn't need to go down with the child every evening. A single kid with a maid plays on her own, and beyond a point there's not much to do, so by the time they are eight or ten, they give up playing. This is especially true of girls. If you have girls who are twelve and above and are actively playing, know that it's time to update your FB status to 'feeling blessed'.

KACCHA LIMBU

Remember the term 'kaccha limbu' — it means that the older kids look after the younger kids. You still get to play with the older kids, you receive the stimuli to run, jump, dodge as fast as the older kids, but all your mistakes are maaf and you are safe. When you grow up and become pakka limbu, you return the favour by looking after other kaccha limbus. If you live within a colony, complex, society that has many kids, handhold the older ones (ten and above, and remember that they are still small themselves, so be gentle) into adopting the kaccha limbu policy. Maybe the adults would need to meet up for a game (hopefully you all have decent fitness levels) — let these kids be a part of it; allow them the experience of a kaccha limbu so that they can look after yours in return.

What should parents do?

You would have figured by now that the theme of this book is for parents to lead by example, especially when it concerns the health of their children. So, here are the **top five guidelines** that you should adopt as parents if you want your children to play / pursue fitness:

1. *Make exercise a non-negotiable part of your life.* Like i have said earlier, and like you already know, kids watch more than they listen. So, exercise for a minimum 150 minutes every week. While you are at it, also read my book *Don't Lose Out, Work Out,* so that you know how to plan your routine. Make it a non-negotiable part of life. And please don't put up statuses of how much you climbed or lifted or ran; treat fitness as a normal, basic requirement of life. And definitely don't come home and tell the kids what daddy or mommy did in the gym, court or grounds today. No one wants to know and they for sure don't want to know. You will look it, smell it, behave it; that's the dignity you should accord your fitness routine. Don't talk about it, chalega?

Coming back to exercise — first, this helps you stay fit yourself, which in the long run is essential for the health of your children. i mean, no one is more stressed than the thirty-year-old who needs to take daddy or mommy for dialysis, sign waivers for bypass, or take chutti for knee replacement. So think long term and invest in your long-term health now. Your kids will value it multi-fold for years to come.

Secondly, fitness or health is a culture that runs in families, even communities. Parents who invest in staying fit also tend to eat, drink, live in a manner that is healthier than those who don't. This has a direct and sustained effect on the health of your children. So, as a household, if you practise eating dinner early, children follow without much resistance. If you wake up early, they do the same; the reverse is true, too.

Even though both parents should be responsible, studies like I.Family prove that the mother's behaviour, her eating habits and lifestyle have a much bigger effect on kids than that of the father. In my line of work, if i work with a mother, i hardly ever end up working with her children, but she will always report that 'the kids are also now eating exactly like me'. But a lot of my kiddie clients have been sent to me by their fathers. Typically, because a father's behaviour doesn't influence the kid much, they have to invest extra money and send the kid to the same dietitian; i mean, i am not complaining — i love the work, i love the daddies and i love the kiddies.

CHILDREN AND EXERCISE SCIENCE

There are many ways in which our muscles produce energy; broadly they are defined as Type 1 and Type

2. Type 1 is slow movement, longer bouts, sustained energy. Type 2 is fast movement, short bouts, powerful energy. So a sprint would be Type 2 and a marathon, Type 1. Children are naturally Type 2 dominant, so while they will excel in sprints, jumps, frog jumps, etc., they get bored with longer runs, like running around a court, ground or running a marathon. And yes, adults are more Type 1, so find it difficult to run up stairs or sprint or do jumps, but can do marathons, long walks, long bouts of cycling with relative ease. And if you force your children to do long-lasting or Type 1-dominating activities, then it will deplete them of the natural Type 2 advantage, so don't do that. So, if you are a marathon-running parent, please don't subject your child to running the marathon; instead, use her like a water girl. She can sprint between you and your running mates, offering water, feeling useful and on top of the world. Also, if you are a coach, devise ways to teach them warm-ups that are skill-specific, and not the generic 'run five rounds of the ground' type, or else they are quick to lose interest in the game.

2. *Once a week, walk with them to school.* Fitness has to be intricately woven into our lifestyle, and movement is one of the best ways of making it happen. Long after you are gone,

your child will remember walking to or back from school with you every Wednesday. It's the things that you watch together, say to each other and moments that you spend with each other that make life as beautiful as it's meant to be. If school is very far away, park a kilometre away and walk once a week, or cycle together, your choice, but teach kids that cities and towns where one can walk are something that we need to work towards. If you are able to get this adopted in the PTA, it will even build political pressure to make roads near schools safe and pedestrian-friendly. If not to school, then to the market or to a friend's place, but move together on foot in a non-competitive manner; build that routine.

i would go to the extent of saying, choose a home for your family where there is plenty of access to open spaces. Of both kinds — public parks and inside your compound — so that there's plenty of stimuli to move, run, jump, everything. Basically, this means if you have to choose between an extra bedroom and access to open spaces with kids playing freely, pick the latter, ankh band karke. It's really not about extra room, extra leg space, etc.; it's about excess baggage, and kids are going to carry that if your house upgrade comes at the cost of play time, company and access to open spaces. High body fat levels in children under ten are associated with a risk to developing cardiovascular disease and cancer as adults. The leaner they are, the better protected they are from diseases. Invest your money in keeping them mobile.

THINK GLOBAL, ACT LOCAL

Ideally, as we get more global, we should want much more than to just sip martinis on the terrace of our new three BHK. With better access to everything that's happening around the globe, we must realise that politics and power struggles are the same everywhere, but living in a democracy means that we, the people, can be the lever of change. This is where we must take inspiration from Americans, in the way they participate in their democracy, not in what they are eating for breakfast, please. Regular people are active in politics; they decide whether a bar or a petrol pump can be set up in their locality, they make themselves heard. Their politicians and police are exactly like us, maybe even worse, but their people are better than us in demanding and actively seeking more accountability from those in power. We must learn from them and actively lobby for better roads, footpaths, air quality and mass transport. These are the things that affect each one of us, across gender, class and caste divides.

All is not grim even in this regard, though. A large factor in the success of polio eradication in India

> has been the Rotary club. These were regular people who dedicated themselves or at least their Sundays to a better cause. They actively and persistently contributed and ensured that the program met with success. So, in a democracy, we must work with the government and make them work for us.

3. *Don't make their love for sports your business.* Enjoy the game — that's all you should be saying to your child, and mean it. They don't need to be the next Sachin, Saina, Sania, whatever. And don't put your own life on hold for their sports, because once you do that, it builds pressure on them. Not to play but to perform. And once a sport becomes about winning / performing, it loses its sheen. The whole purpose of sport is to feel competitive, play at your best and to be able to enjoy even the way your opponent plays. One of my clients once told me that he went to watch his daughter at a swimming competition; he said all the girls were so good, they finished their swim, picked up their own towel and dried their heads and bodies. My client sat there with stars in his eyes for his little thirteen-year-old; she pretended not to see him. On the other hand, he said, after the boy's event, mommies rushed to the finish line and wiped their heads with dry towels — this was an under-fifteen tournament. My client's heart broke, and he

said, which jerk will my daughter date? So watch, but from a distance, and watch only sometimes, not all tournaments, and no fussing. If it's not making them self-sufficient, it's not worth the money, time or stars in the eyes.

4. *Take holidays that keep you mobile once every year.* And i don't mean walking around in a mall. Trek to the Himalaya or the Sahyadris. Take a rafting trip, sign up on a cycling holiday, take skiing lessons together. Essentially, take holidays where you will be moving physically, where the network won't work and where there won't be anything to buy. That's when you will learn to depend on each other, push each other to do better, and you can watch your child finish everything on the plate without complaints. When one is physically out of one's comfort zone is when the feel-good hormones are released. If you have a little tot, a holiday like this is your chance to build a rich and diverse gut bacteria environment. If it's an eight- to twelve-year-old, it's your chance to have them explore how communities live in tune with nature, how animals are a part of farms and families. And if it's a teenager, the best chance to get to know them, and when their chances of sharing secrets with you are heightened. More under the 'Holidays' section in Part 2 of the book.

5. *Don't stop them from playing because of the weather.* Too many kids have been kept away from playing because it is either raining, too hot, too cold, etc. Weather conditions are natural and recurring, and if you allow them, kids will

find a way to play things that are weather-suitable. E.g., cricket in the summer, football in the rains. If you keep them indoors due to the weather, the only way they will stay entertained is with a gadget: TV, iPad and the likes. And then the more they watch TV, the more they demand junk food. The I.Family project has shown that there is a clustering of lifestyle behaviours: watching the screen (irrespective of the duration) increases children's demand for SSB (sugar-sweetened beverages) in particular (colas, caffeinated energy drinks, juices, etc.) and junk food in general. So this whole sit at home because it's too cold / too hot is not just preventing them from getting the benefits of playing outdoors but also exposing them to the dangers of junk food. Also, please, it hurts me to say this, but don't stop your girls from swimming or being out in the afternoon in the fear ke rang kala ho jayega. Please, for heaven's sake, the world is not a happier or kinder place if you are as fair as you can be, but if you are as strong and self-reliant as you can be. Bolu kya wapas ke samajh gaya? And no, don't stop your boys for things like oh the mosquitoes will bite, the grass is too tall, the floor is too slippery. We need strong boys too, not needy, dependent ones, please.

Essentially, build the fitness and health narrative beyond 'how do i look', 'what size am i fitting in', 'what is my weight / height'. Create opportunities for them to explore the many benefits of staying fit in a wholesome manner. Good health is the foundation to growth, transformation, exploration, to learning, to leading a good, fun, wholesome life. Don't let it get limited to aesthetics only. When you lead a good life, it shows on you, but that's not the point of it. Live it so that your children know it.

And yes, don't forget activity. That's much more crucial than exercise in the long term. Do things at home by yourself. Once a week, wash your own clothes or sweep your room or clean the fans — it will make you look cooler than you are. Make your own bed every day, pick your own coffee, chai cup and those of others around you. Don't make the driver come up with your bag, carry it yourself, it's not going to break your back. A moving home is a happy home. A happy home is a healthy home. Being a man of the house is not a license to lounge, and if you do belong to that kind of thinking, know that lifestyle diseases are walking closer to you by the minute.

Important note: Sharing our open spaces

All genders need support and access to open places if they must reap the benefit of good health and grow optimally. Kids who are underprivileged need it even more. For all our global citizen giri, liberal mind-set, etc., if there's a slum kid next to our child at the park, we will get restless. Well, it's ok to feel restless, but you must reassure yourself that a free and fair world means equal access to everyone, especially with regard to public spaces. We must encourage that wholeheartedly and overcome our biases and prejudices. Recently, the rich neighbourhood of Malabar Hill in Mumbai wanted to deny slum kids access to a park. Well, the same people have their faces flashed in fashion magazines for their charities for the poor. But dahling, charity begins with sharing open spaces and teaching your kids to wait their turn for the swing.

While at it, the one issue that needs our attention is girls in open spaces or public parks. All the big maidans are monopolised by boys, and while at home and school, we must individually teach them to be more inclusive and share open spaces with girls; **we must also work at reserving days or ear-marking areas for girls to play.** i mean, i really don't care about women's reservation in Parliament because so many times it just means that biwi, beti, bahu, bhabi will occupy the seat. The real Bharat needs reservation of open spaces for girls and at least for three to five years for it to be effective. Change is slow, and the first day you reserve the space, all won't come out and play; it takes time. You know, in politics we will argue, give the government at least five years — same thing in play, give our girls at least five years. And then you mark my words, Indian girls will do well in team sports too, not just in individual sports.

LONG-TERM WEIGHT LOSS

You know, i am treading on eggshells here, but hear me out. A lot of women want to reinvent themselves, especially post childbirth, and somehow shedding weight is the most accepted or popular way to do it. Even within that, being on an extreme diet, only keto, only protein, only salad, only whatever, seems to be the rule to do it. The thing is that torture or deprivation never led to health or happiness for anyone and it won't be the case with you either. Your best case scenario is that you will be thin for a couple of weeks and back to being bloated, constipated or plain fat in the next few weeks. Losing weight will seem like a constant struggle or the most dominant conversation, thought and action. Now this, of course, creates an extremely unhealthy role model for your child, especially the girl child. But what you must know is that you didn't get out of shape all of a sudden. We all like to blame it on shaadi, kaam and bachhe, but look deeper and the real reason is because you were not optimally active or playing as hard as you should have between the ages of zero and fifteen years. You could have done that to be girly then — you are probably killing yourself trying to lose weight to look girly now — but just imagine how much you will ruin the life of your daughter if she inherits these concepts of being girly. Strong, self-reliant, seeking no approval is what she should be inheriting, but she will inherit that from your actions not words or books, so watch out.

And no, all is not lost if you were not active then; start now and start slow, one step at a time and make it into a sustainable lifestyle that leads to long-term weight loss. Recognise that you have been out of shape for ten to fifteen years, you may have noticed it only now, but then take your time to lose it. Even if you lose it in the next three years, at least it's gone permanently and your daughter has not inherited body shaming or self-consciousness — isn't that a great deal?

Typically, done right and sustainably (not obsessively):

- Fit for ten years before childbirth: back in shape in the range of six to nine weeks.
- Out of shape for the last five years: about nine to twelve months to get back in shape.
- Hostel and courses like engineering, architecture, medicine, law: two to three years.
- IVF: add one more year to the above.

5 EXERCISE GUIDELINES FOR PARENTS

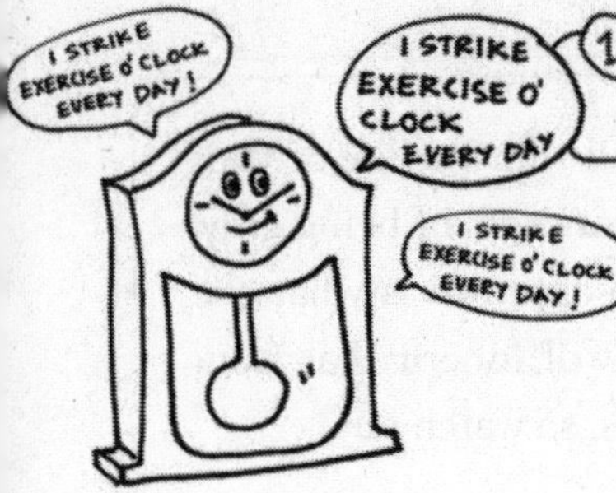

1. MAKE EXERCISE A NON-NEGOTIABLE PART OF YOUR LIFE

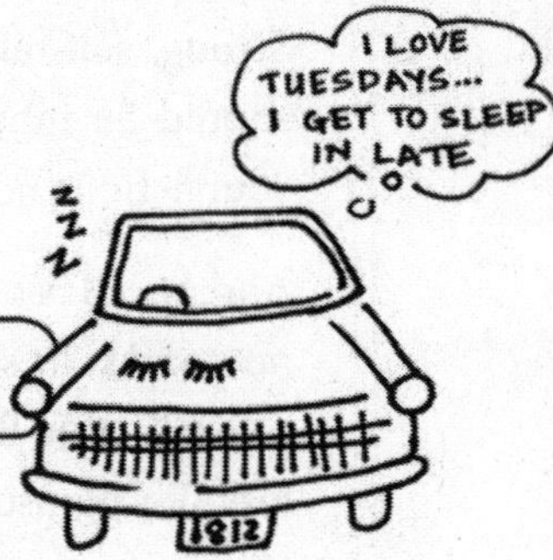

2. ONCE A WEEK, WALK WITH THEM TO SCHOOL

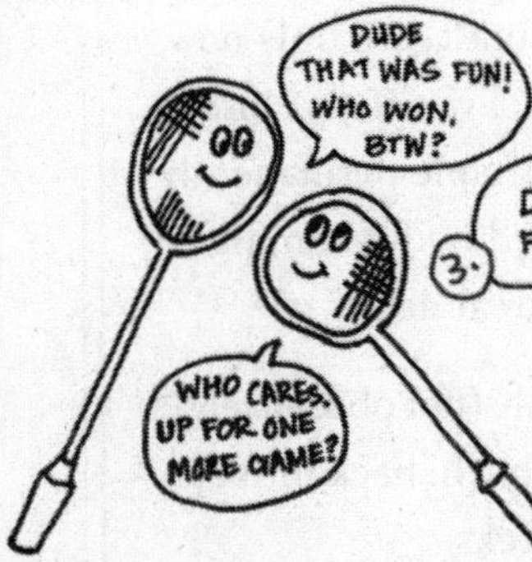

3. DON'T MAKE THEIR LOVE FOR SPORT YOUR BUSINESS

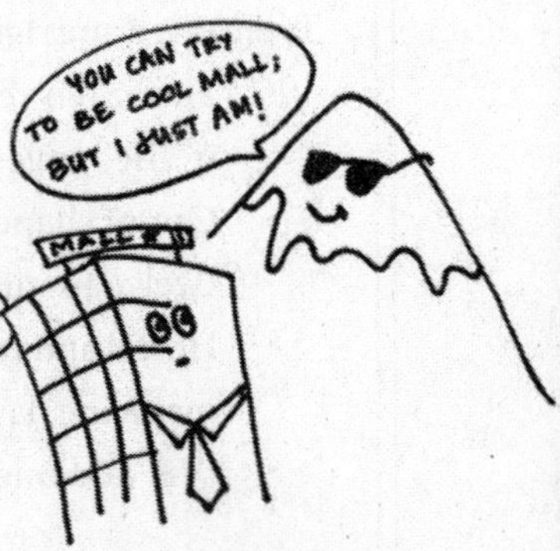

4. ACTIVE HOLIDAYS ONCE A YEAR

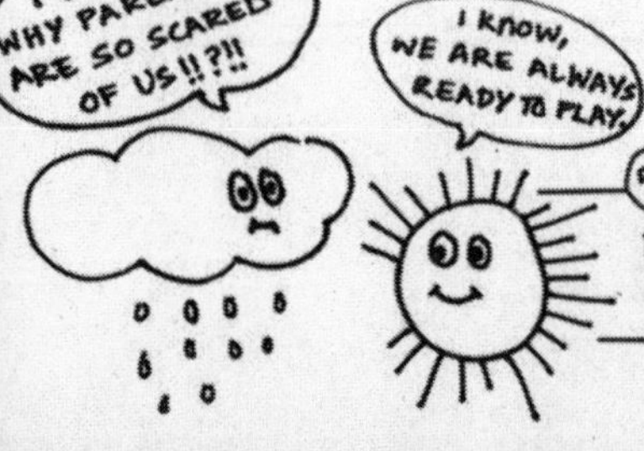

5. DON'T STOP THEM FROM PLAYING BECAUSE OF THE WEATHER

Chapter 4

For Kids — Keep Moving

Childhood is defined by bodies that move at a fast pace and minds that stay still, focused. The persistency with which children chase their curiosity is a sign of wisdom; so is the pace and grace with which they move their bodies. Now, instead of nurturing these beautiful traits, we adults want to tame them. We tame the curiosity and the speed. We duck questions, warn them about running too fast. Schools punish kids for running in corridors. i hope that, with time, adults will mature and understand that what defines childhood should be celebrated, not suppressed. But till then, here's what you kids can do to fight us stupid, old adults.

FIVE THINGS KIDS SHOULD DO TO STAY FIT

1. Learn a balancing movement, like cycling, skating, skiing, gymnastics

When you went from being practically immobile to

slipping, it was progress. Then you worked hard to first raise your head and stabilise (the head is heavy, so well done), then lift your upper body on fully stretched arms, then up went the hip, and finally the whole lower body on your knees. Before you learned to crawl, you learned to stabilise your spine. Once stabilised, mobility is easy, graceful and delightful. Basically, if you have made it here, you can make it anywhere. From thereon, walking and running is a cakewalk; all that you had to do was distribute your weight equally on your two feet.

Now you must take it a notch higher and continue building on the kinaesthetic intelligence of your young body. What better way than to learn the balancing acts — skating, cycling, skiing, gymnastics? You know, movement is probably the most critical aspect of human life. Being in a war-torn country, and in some cases just belonging to the female gender, feels like punishment, because free movement is restricted. On the other hand, when we began crawling is also when we began talking. Language is one of the most complex of human tasks and it is movement that makes it possible. So work at investing at least three to four hours every week in a balancing act; it will give you an immense sense of power, freedom and intelligence, both to the body and the brain.

IS IT OK TO GYM?

Yes, is the short answer. You can gym from any age, surely from fifteen but even from eight, if you have found yourself a good trainer. A good trainer is one who understands exercise physiology, kinesiology and bio-mechanics (these are basic subjects of exercise, sport and movement), and who knows about and practises the specifics of the Adolescent Training Program (ATP).

You can gym once a week or thirty to forty-five minutes a week, along with everything else that you are doing. The one thing that you should be aware of is 'failure'. This occurs when you cannot do another repetition in strict form; your trainer understands this. So lift weight that doesn't take you to failure till you are eighteen or even twenty-one. As an adult, though, you should hit failure in the gym. A child's body grows without the stimuli of failure; an adult's body needs failure to respond or adapt to stimuli.

And it's a myth that gymming affects your growth and keeps you short, it doesn't. Nor does cycling or basketball increase your height. This is called as reverse selection of sport. Professional basketball is dominated by tall individuals and power-lifting by short ones, as height or lack of it gives them an edge in their preferred sport. Both have to gym, though, to get better at their sport and to prevent injuries.

2. *Yogasanas are great for kids, but not meditation or pranayama*

Actually, yoga was inspired by nature, by trees, rivers, mountains, peacocks, lions and little children. So children don't really need to learn yoga; yoga has learnt from them. Mostly about keeping the body laghu or light, and the mind open and curious.

But if you must go to a class, or if you are being taught yoga in school, then know that it should 90 per cent be all about asanas, bodily movement. There could be a short prayer, but beyond that it shouldn't require you to sit in one place and just breathe or meditate.

When Patanjali (the saint who lived around 5,000 years ago, and probably contributed the most to yoga in India and should not be confused with products that Baba Ramdev sells) wrote down the best practices from across all yoga schools, he gave the study of yoga a structure. That structure is called as Ashtanga, the eight steps or limbs of yoga. According to that, the first three steps —

yama, niyama, asana — you must practise and do daily; the rest — pranayama, pratyahar, dhyan, dharana, samadhi — happen. Yama is self-restraint, so not hitting someone even when you feel like it is yama; you must practice it. Niyama is rules — reaching class on time, finishing assignments on time are rules set by school; you must follow those too. Asanas use the body to create all that we see in nature: to be inspired by the mountain to be tall, to create right angles like a triangle, etc.; these, too, you must do.

The rest is not for doing, or at least shouldn't be more than 10 per cent of your class (higher side). The business and popularity of yoga means that there are too many teachers and they may be in a rush to get you to stages beyond the first three. But these cannot be taught, much less practised by kids. So keep it simple, and my recommendation is five suryanamaskars every day after the age of seven years for every child. It consists of a sequence of twelve asanas, done on both sides of the body: the prefect recipe for mobility, agility and stability. Especially important if you play any sport, particularly racquet sports. You can see a video of suryanamaskar here — https://goo.gl/2FgYAu

3. Choose play over studies any day

i mean, this one is very simple, isn't it? Too many kids have given up on playing because they are in 10th, 12th or whatever, but it's not worth it at all. While education is important, all-round education is even more important. Your marks are surely not a sign of how bright or dull you are, but your lethargy will tell on you and your life scores soon. So, no matter what, choose the daily dose of free play over everything — tuition class, revision, completing homework, everything. In the long run, this is what matters. Free play is fuelling growth of every cell in your body, brain and being — don't lose out on that for some impermanent, fleeting glory like stars on the hand, coming first in class or whatever.

4. Learn at least one classical instrument or dance

Ah! This is much more important than i can ever explain. When you learn a classical art form, you learn the ability to see music and hear colours. Now you have to experience this, and all it will take is the investment of two to three hours a week over three to five years. It wires your brain differently and you are then able to see stability or steadiness in movement and hear silence in between words, songs and rhythm. It increases the number of nerves per unit of muscle fibre in your body, giving you a lead of at least twenty years in maturity, as compared to anybody else, and paradoxically, twenty years of anti-ageing too. If you look at any classical artist, whether it's Ustad Zakir Hussain, Vyjayanthimala or Pandit Jasraj, they all look at least twenty years younger than anybody of their age, and when they perform, they seem ageless. You can also choose to learn a classical martial art.

5. *Ninety minutes of free play, every day*

You probably got the drift of this earlier also. But you know, thoda nagging banta hai, angrezi mein it's called reaffirming. Anyway, so every day, on the day that you have your most important exam, on the day you are travelling, on the day that someone is coming over (on the day that you get ditched, on the day that you feel all is lost, on the day that you feel like running away from home — all normal emotions, haan, read only if you are above fifteen), no matter what, play. It will keep you happy and give you a sense of being in charge of everything that is happening in your life. It will give your confidence a boost, keep the friendly and diverse communities of bacteria in your stomach and gut thriving, improve blood circulation to every part of your body and brain.

And it should be for sixty minutes at least, ideally ninety minutes, but outdoors, outside of the house, i mean. And anything is ok. Badminton, basketball, lock and key, kabbadi, just running around in your complex, anything is good, but not video games, not board games. Ok? Anything that is short but has repeated bursts of high intensity activity. On a Sunday or weekend, play more, not less. And no, that play area in a mall doesn't count as real play. Do the real thing — sweat, dirt, grime. Ok?

Important note: Stay active, all the time

Activity is different from exercise; it's the day-to-day tasks that you perform that require bodily movement. Walking to school is activity, cleaning your room is activity, washing your plate is activity. Technically, if you look at it, staying active has more heart-protecting benefits than even exercise. Choose opportunities to stay active in your daily life. Whether at home, school, or a community centre — like a place of religious worship, public park, housing society complex — ask what you can do, to be more useful. Childhood, i feel, is the most powerless phase of one's life, as you are dependent for money, safety, food, everything. But with activity, you can help. Kaamave toh saamave, my grandfather, Appa, always told me. Loosely, it means if you are useful, you will always belong.

So, every day, think of what can you do to stay useful. Pick up your clothes, pack your own bag, wash your tiffin box. Make your own bed; jhadu-poocha your room, maybe the home every week; plant a native tree in the building. Help with arrangements of a festival, fair, exhibition; volunteer at your school, community centre ... the list is endless. In your head, you split it in two parts — small stuff that you do daily, big stuff that you do weekly or monthly or as required. When you are a guest in someone's home, do more than what you do in your own home. Eat the food served with love and gratitude, help clean up and set the table, stay useful, in every setting.

You can even learn small cooking tasks, like setting the curd, boiling the milk, making chai (for parents and family only — you stay away from all things caffeine, chai and chocolate), as is age appropriate. Activity is your way to make the world a better place, one task at a time. This is the home-ground of self-reliance, independence and strength, and it's never too early to begin.

OUR WEALTH: THE YOUNG POPULATION

In October 2015, i was sitting in a coffee shop in a beautiful suburb of Berlin, Potsdam. Every morning i would go there to have my coffee before going for my course on 'future foods' at the university. Everything was right out of a picture book — beautiful cafés, footpaths, trams, cycling tracks — but something seemed amiss. Every morning, i would sit by the window, sipping coffee, watching the street and wonder saalaa, kya lafda hai? What is it that doesn't seem right? Then about a week or ten days later, it struck me like a Eureka moment. 'Shit,' i said aloud and smiled. The lafda was that the street scenes were dominated by old people. Well, not geriatric or anything. They were able-bodied, even fit-bodied, but mostly people who looked like they were in their fifties, thirties probably being the youngest. From my office window on Linking Road, Khar, if i look out, at any point i will see at least five young kids and plenty of teenagers and people in their twenties. When i walk home, i see even younger kids: i pass two schools, one dance class and one coffee shop. i mean, i see lots of people in their forties, fifties, even eighties, but the youth dominates the scene. i concluded that Khar is richer than Postdam, because our street scenes have pace, laughter and, very simply, the optimism of youth. Optimism is richness.

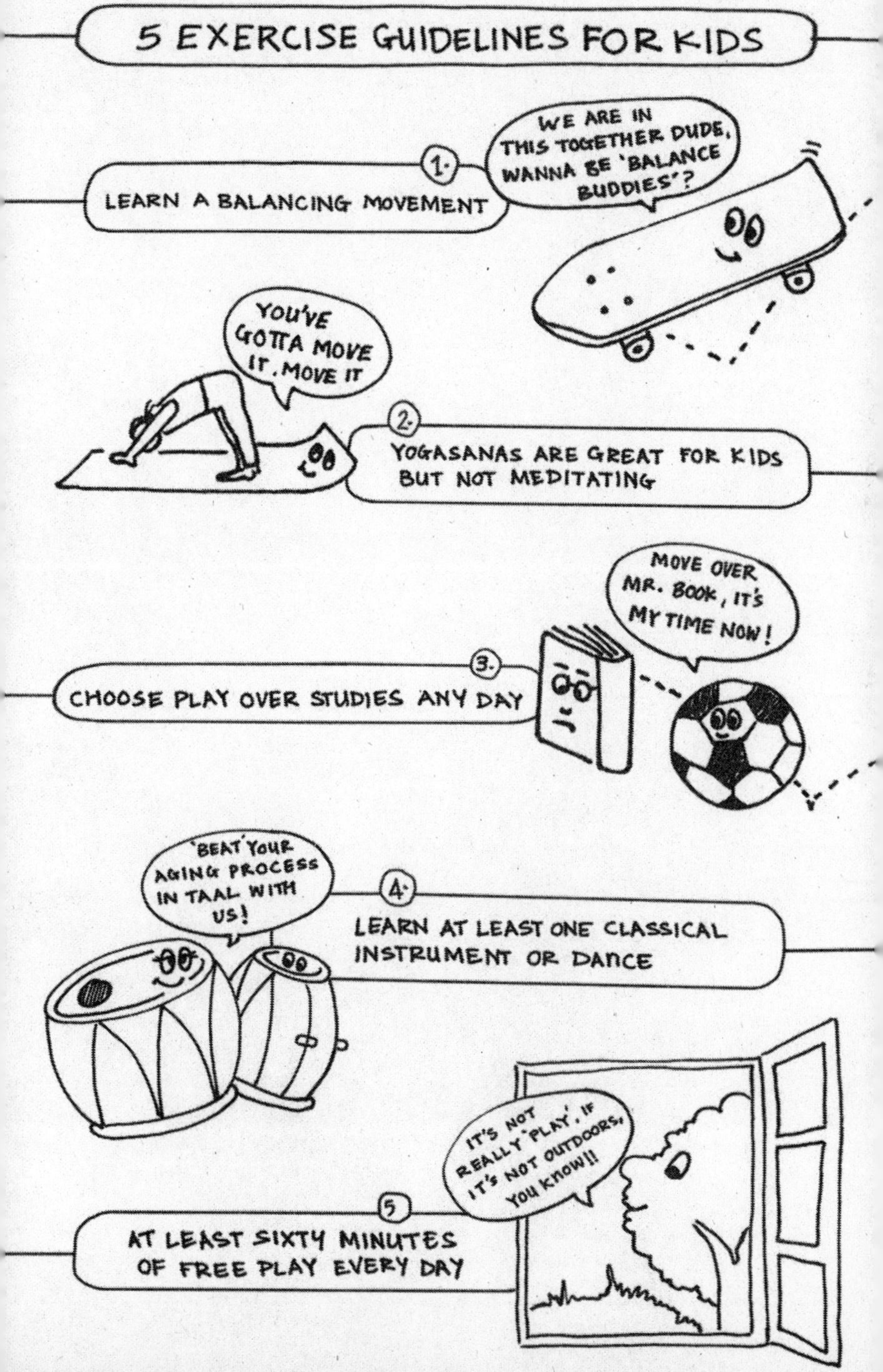
5 EXERCISE GUIDELINES FOR KIDS
1. LEARN A BALANCING MOVEMENT
WE ARE IN THIS TOGETHER DUDE, WANNA BE 'BALANCE BUDDIES'?
YOU'VE GOTTA MOVE IT, MOVE IT
2. YOGASANAS ARE GREAT FOR KIDS BUT NOT MEDITATING
MOVE OVER MR. BOOK, IT'S MY TIME NOW!
3. CHOOSE PLAY OVER STUDIES ANY DAY
'BEAT' YOUR AGING PROCESS IN TAAL WITH US!
4. LEARN AT LEAST ONE CLASSICAL INSTRUMENT OR DANCE
IT'S NOT REALLY 'PLAY', IF IT'S NOT OUTDOORS, YOU KNOW!!
5. AT LEAST SIXTY MINUTES OF FREE PLAY EVERY DAY

PART 2: PRACTICAL APPLICATIONS

Part 2a — Age-Wise

i) Zero to Two Years

The first 1,000 days of life — that's from the time that the woman gets pregnant to the child's second birthday — are considered most important. This is when the brain grows, nutrition foundation is set and a healthy future can be secured. In fact, poor nutrition at this critical stage, zero to two years, can transcend generations and take chronic diseases to future generations as well. This is the MOST important period to future-proof the health and well-being of your child.

The top three Sustainable Development Goals — zero poverty, zero hunger, health and well-being for all — are actually rooted in this time period. Good nourishment at this stage can boost a country's GDP by 12 per cent, prevent millions of deaths and healthcare costs, and most importantly, reduce the disparities between health, education and earning potential. Let's not forget that we as a country are in this unique position of having the most malnourished and second-most number of obese children in the world. So for us, this period is even more critical, and if baby formula has been prescribed to us, then our battle with the bulge has already begun. One that will inflate the industry's bottom line and our child's waistline. What's worse? It doesn't allow for the gut microbiota diversity that would otherwise blossom if we simply ate according to our food heritage. So, here is looking at the three most important foods for the infant.

But first things first, breastfeed and exclusively for the first six months of the baby's life. There is no equivalent to breast milk. i can't emphasise this enough, and you can read the following recommendation by WHO and UNICEF:

To enable mothers to establish and sustain exclusive breastfeeding for six months, WHO and UNICEF recommend:

- *Initiation of breastfeeding within the first hour of life;*
- *Exclusive breastfeeding — that is, the infant only receives breastmilk without any additional food or drink, not even water;*
- *Breastfeeding on demand — that is, as often as the child wants, day and night;*
- *No use of bottles, teats or pacifiers.*

Breastmilk is the natural first food for babies; it provides all the energy and nutrients that the infant needs for the first months of life, and it continues to provide up to half or more of a child's nutritional needs during the second half of the first year, and up to one-third during the second year of life.

*Breastfeeding contributes to the health and well-being of mothers, it helps to space children, reduces the risk of ovarian cancer and breast cancer, increases family and national resources, is a secure way of feeding and is safe for the environment.**

So here we go: **top three foods for age group zero to two years:**

1. Desi cow milk: If you fall short of breastmilk supply or choose not to breastfeed for some reason, the second-best option is desi cow milk. Desi cow milk is easy to digest, provides the new baby with diverse and gut-friendly microbes, along with essential vitamins, minerals and proteins.

It's important, however, to dilute the milk with water and to add a herb called vavding to it. This is available in any trusted Ayurvedic shop and your grandmom may even have it stored safely in her kitchen or batwa; talk to her. This tiny spice doesn't just protect the kid from developing infections and diseases, but also makes digestion easy and is especially useful in colicky kids or those that are troubled with too much gas. It's also known by the name of 'false pepper'.

It's unfortunate that in a country where indigenous

---

* http://www.who.int/nutrition/topics/exclusive_breastfeeding/en/

wisdom about the best first food is freely available, the prescription is often infant formulas. In fact, a lot of hospitals give formula milk as the first feed even before breastmilk. That infant formulas are high on cheap sugars, low on nourishment and do not allow for diversity of friendly microbes is well known, yet no one bats an eyelid before prescribing it, and we don't think that there's anything wrong in buying it either. In the Philippines, there was an uproar recently against paediatric clinics having pictures of infant formula on their walls, and for insisting on formula milk as the preferred feed. In India, too, banned substances like GMOs were found in formulas that were prescribed to kids who had a lot of allergies. i desperately want to believe that Indian doctors are not doing this for the kickbacks from food companies, but only because of nutritionism that is entrenched in their education system. As far as we, the regular people, are concerned, we should opt for shudh desi versions of first foods that have stood the test of time over anything industrialised, mass-produced and advertised.

DESI COWS

India, as a developing economy, is at a place where it is still not so difficult to raise a cow of your own.

No, seriously. Our Tier 2 and Tier 3 cities still have the option of owning a small patch of green without it costing the moon. Then to get a desi cow is a one-time investment. But ensure that you pay the person who looks after her well, because tending to a cow and knowing how and when to milk her is a special skill. If people with the ability to pay get kanjus about this, then in the long term this will become a lost art. For all of us who are in villages and have cows, we must know that we are really fortunate to have the ability to raise a free-roaming, grass-grazing cow. And that this is a matter of great pride; in terms of health, it's better than owning a luxury car.

In fact, now there are quite a few IIT-IIM types who see this as a gold mine and far more stimulating than the jobs or money that big companies can offer them. And then there is that added advantage of the good karma that anything health-related brings, especially if you do a good job with it. All that the desi cow milk needs is positioning and packaging as the best first food for babies, because it really is, and well, yes, it needs freedom from the political positioning.

As for all of you who are worried about the hormones in milk and cruelty towards the calf, buy from small farms who look after their cows. And if we had been taught about farming and the basics of agriculture in school, then we would know that if the calf drinks all the milk that the cow produces, it could actually harm him. If you ever visit a farm and observe while a calf drinks off the mother, after a while the cow will push the calf away. This is simply to protect the calf. When it comes to a lactating cow, it's always two udders for the calf and two for the farmer's family; the kids will even drink it straight from the udders. This was, and is, a non-cruel, non-harming method for all involved. Indian and African communities knew a thing or two about sustainability long before the word was invented. The 'untouched by hand' milk comes from all four udders, so your 'hygiene' is coming at the cost of cruelty to the animal.

How to feed: Avoid the bottle and that plastic nipple. In Indian households, you have this tiny little baby-specific utensil called bondla or paladai. It's basically a broad, shallow cup, with a handle on one side and a long groove-like spout, a little like a cut open tube, on the other. Often made of silver or brass, the practice is to take the milk in the shallow part, blow on it to cool it, put the spout by the corner of the baby's lips and pour a little at a time. Want to know the preferred position to do so? The grandmom or the older aunt often sits with her legs outstretched in the dandasana position, the baby is kept with her head by the woman's feet and toes towards her knees. Then the woman bends over with an open chest and a straight spine and pours a little milk, a few drops at a time, into the baby's mouth. In the times of Instagram, it may not get many likes, but all it needs is one Western university to show how this practice is healthy, constitutes for safe feeding, gives the new mother a chance to relax and for the baby to bond with other members of the family, and this little piece will sell like hot cakes. Dr Raghunath Mashelkar may have to fight off patenting efforts just like he fought for turmeric and Basmati rice not to be patented. But once this is done, Indians will buy it, like the way we buy the squatty potty now.

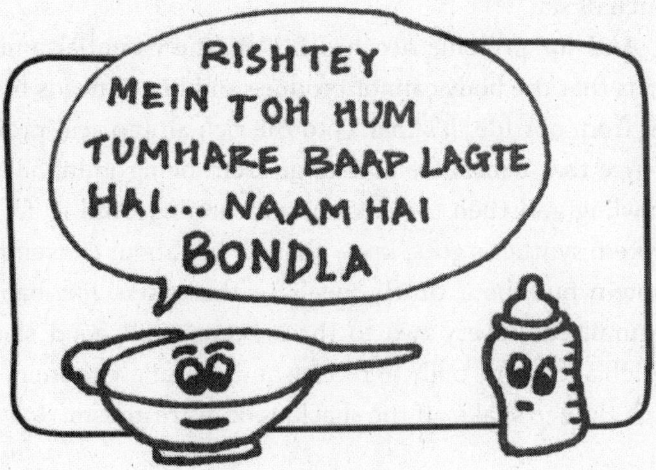
RISHTEY MEIN TOH HUM TUMHARE BAAP LAGTE HAI... NAAM HAI BONDLA

2. Rice porridge: Oh! For all those who think of rice as only carb or starch or empty calories, i have got news. Rice has been one of our first foods since centuries, and Bill Aitken, the living legend of Himalayan exploration, often says that people have not been doing things for centuries for nothing (this he said to me to protest the Indian government's plan to open the chardham yatra for twelve months a year, when for centuries it has been opened only during the summer months). So why rice? Well, for starters, it's easy on the stomach and light to digest. More importantly, it has resistant starch that works as a prebiotic, which is food for probiotics or the good bacteria. And at six months is when the bacterial diversity begins to bloom in the baby's little gut, in her entire body, in fact, and what better than rice to fuel that growth? Easy to cook, easy to digest and great to taste, add just a dollop of ghee and a pinch of salt.

And for protein, rice has BCAA, the essential amino acids that the body cannot produce and hence needs to be fed from outside. It's thanks to the rich amino acid profile of rice that babies are able to go from being immobile to crawling and then to walking and running. And as far as protein synthesis goes, know that it's not about consuming protein but about timely meals (eating often, like babies naturally do, every two to three hours) and good sleep, which allows the body to receive and assimilate protein. So high time to shake off the shackles of nutritionism.

Ragi satva or ragi porridge is as popular as rice porridge. The key is to make both into a thin slurry, not watery, like the consistency of fresh paint. Then, as the child grows, you reduce the amount of water you are adding to the rice and start adding just a little bit of dal. In some communities, they just add dal ka pani to rice porridge, instead of dal.

How to feed: Rice, in fact rice kheer, is one of the meals that the child's maternal uncle feeds her during ushtavan or annaprashan, the ceremony that takes place when the baby turns six months old. This is often served on a little silver plate or bowl and then fed with the hands (no nail polish or long nails, please) to the baby. Silver, as you are aware, works as a natural antibacterial and antiviral agent, and feeding babies on silverware ensures that you can ward off infections and the barrage of antibiotics that get prescribed with it. It breaks my heart that so many Indian kids have been on more than one antibiotic dose even before they turn two. This, when it is well known that losing gut flora at this stage is going to be so dangerous for them in the long term. It puts their hormones at risk, can mess up their metabolism, sleep cycle, just about everything that would secure a healthy future for them. So, stay off the plastic stuff, be it sippers, bowls, spoons, and go back to your traditions. A healthy future is priceless and worth fighting for, even if it makes you look not with it, while you are at it.

3. Banana: Officially our first fruit. Again, a prebiotic, a stomach-soother, a complete meal by itself. If you look at all the nutrients it offers, it's like taking a multivitamin syrup. Especially useful when the baby is travelling or when you are taking her to someone's home where you are not sure if they will be kind and thoughtful enough to make khichdi or some rice for your child. The banana is so good that it could be all — breakfast, lunch or dinner — to your child. Especially when they are feeling low or recovering from a flu and the appetite is not fully back.

How to feed: Peel the banana just before you are about to feed the baby. Not fully, just as much as you need, and limit exposure of the rest of the banana to air so that it doesn't begin to oxidise and lose its nutrient value. Remember, kids eat slowly, so don't rush them. Instead be patient and artist-like with peeling the banana. Then take off a bit of the banana, mash it in between your fingers, and feed it with your hands to the baby. Don't force the baby to finish the full banana; go with the flow. Big or small, any banana is ok, but keep it local.

To summarise, this is a critical age. Not only must you avoid industrialised and mass-produced but avoid everything that has no history of being used as baby food in your culture or heritage. Before you feed your baby broccoli, oats and kale, ask yourself if you were fed those as a child. Banana, vavding, bondal, ragi or rice porridge, the ritual of presenting the silver thali to a child may never make it to our textbooks, Instagram or get endorsed by celebs or associations of doctors or dietitians, but that doesn't make them unworthy. They are undervalued because they belong to collective wisdom and since that is nobody's property, it remains an entity that cannot be monetised. That is all that you need to know as far as the question of recommendations go. The industry influence over influencers is huge, but don't let that come in the way of common sense or in the way of valuing and adopting timeless practices.

SWADDLING CLASSES IN THE US

While we give up on our indigenous wisdom of tying up our infants in special malmal cloths, the US goes for special swaddling classes, where new parents learn to do the exact same thing. i could swaddle my younger cousins by the time i was ten years old. i was raised to be useful and to return favours; it's one of the things you learn living in big families. But the thing is, paediatricians are against it, so we give it up. Btw, they are also against rice pej and in favour of formula. My friend, who has a seven-year-old daughter, was advised by her paediatrician to not put her in Bharatnatyam class as that would give her wide hips or even malkhamb, as that would make her short. Well, i cannot even begin to talk about how misplaced this kind of advice is but all that i will say is that if your paediatrician or any doctor or health professional has contempt for time-tested, indigenous practices, it's time to change the doctor.

Eating with hands, speaking in mother tongue, immersing oneself in regional culture is the stuff that makes life rich and moments priceless. If we give up on these now, sometime in the future our kids will be attending how to eat by hand classes, downloading apps that teach them how to say hello and thank you in their mother tongue or going on cultural tours where they are charged fifty dollars an hour to learn rangoli or lejhim. We can't wait for research or foreign press to catch up with basic truths of life. We must continue with them because the proof, really, is in practice.

ii) Two to Five Years

The wonder years, where you can actually enjoy the child the most. Well, actually, not true. You can enjoy them and suffer them at all ages. But this is also the age where they naturally begin to experiment with food and develop a taste for or preferences that may be different from the rest of the family. It is therefore important that they learn that what is good is what is rare, comes once in a while during the season and is unique to their region, community and culture. What is good is what is local, not mass-produced and coming out of a box. What is good is what has been enjoyed for centuries, and which boosts health, local economy and ecology. They are going to be watching you, so what you eat will also begin to make a difference from now on. So, basic question, are you still eating 'protein' for dinner, or have you switched to eating a 'meal' or 'food' for dinner?

Pancha varsha ni lalayat, goes a subhashit, which means that you should indulge kids till they are five. The key is to indulge them with the good stuff, valuable stuff that will bring them health, harmony and happiness in the long term.

Top three foods for age group two–five years:

1. **Jaggery and ghee with roti or bhakri**: This is the best age group in which to introduce this meal. It's a no-fuss, dry and easy-to-carry meal, be it to school, playgrounds or on long journeys. This is the right age group for your child to watch and learn how roti or bhakri is broken into tiny pieces with one hand and mixed with jaggery and gul, using the same hand. The millet bhakri or the wheat roti that you use will bring in its own nutrient profile, but the ghee and jaggery mixture here is the real hero. It soothes and smoothens the digestive processes, provides the body with iron and folate and gives a boost to the immune system. If you live in a place with extreme heat, replace jaggery with sugar for that season.

These days, a lot of parents write to me asking what they can do to ensure that their two- or three-year-old is not constipated. They are often prescribed a laxative or a fibre drink and oats for breakfast or fruits to add more fibre to the diet. But the thing is, if you do add so much fibre to the child's diet, they are going to drop low on their mineral assimilation, especially iron and calcium. This is the age group that they start hopping, running, sprinting and they need the calcium to keep the bones strong and muscles agile. This is also the age group where, if you make nutrient-based choices, they will fall short of iron, get anaemic and then fall sick with every change of weather or even mood. The key is to think big, look towards your food heritage and pick an option that's tasty to eat, provides a rich nutrient profile, not just one or two nutrients, and makes for a no-fuss meal. The roti-jaggery-ghee will prevent constipation and can be eaten well into adulthood too, and — at this stage — makes for a good lunch or a wholesome snack option. Even dinner, if they don't fancy what has been cooked.

How to feed: First, sit on the floor. Take the silver thali, put the fresh roti or bhakri in the centre and ghee and jaggery on the side. Mix ghee and jaggery to a jam-like consistency. If you are using a millet, add a little extra ghee, especially if it's bajra or makai. Then break the roti into tiny pieces, mix it in the ghee and jaggery, the way you would mix it in sabzi, and feed it to the child. As the kid grows up, break the roti into tiny pieces and encourage her to eat on her own. As they grow even bigger, teach them to break the roti on their own with just one hand. It improves neuro muscular coordination and teaches them to manipulate objects easily.

Also, culturally, we eat with one hand, the right one preferably. You all know what the left one is for — washing after the big job. And the other job of the left hand is also to serve yourself from common vessels. In terms of yoga, it is about keeping the prana and the apana in a state of balance so as to optimise the sammana, the energy used for digestion. If you spend a million dollars and go for an Ayurvedic nutrition workshop at a spa in Austria or upstate New York, this is what they will teach you — or you can learn it for free at home.

2. Metkut: A combination of dals and spices like haldi, made into a powder (like a dry chutney), and mixed with rice and had as lunch or dinner. You can expect the child to go off dal anytime now and, as discussed earlier, it's because of the naturally existing anti-nutrients in there. The stomach is still small right now, and though it needs the amino acid profile from dals and pulses, it needs to come in a way where the trypsin inhibitors don't hurt the protein assimilation processes of the body. Lo and behold, your grandma has made you metkut. Made in a way that keeps the anti-nutrients down, provides a good nutrient profile and still keeps the meal no-fuss and tasty.

METKUT RECIPE

2 katori chana dal

1 katori raw rice

½ katori poha

2 tsp of dhania

1 tsp jeera

A few red chillies

Khada hing

- Dry roast all together and then grind to a fine powder.

- Add a tsp to steam rice with a tsp of ghee, mix well and eat.

Happy meals are made of thee.

How to feed: Mix a teaspoon of metkut in hot, freshly prepared rice and then add a dollop of ghee and salt to taste. The key here is good mixing, so mash the rice well. It all needs to look like a uniform mixture where you can't tell the rice from the metkut or the ghee. Then make small bites, mash it a little more in your hands and feed the child while she sits cross-legged on the floor. As she grows up, make tiny balls of metkut bhat and place them a little away from each other, so that the growing child has enough room to put her tiny fingers around these mounds of rice and pick them up — using only one hand, of course, and encourage them to take their time. There is no rush to get them to eat as quickly as possible. This is often the age group where we begin to chide them to quickly finish a meal, and in the process have large molecules of food entering their stomachs, leading to weak digestion. Since this is the age group where they pick and learn instinctively, teach them to chew slowly, on all sides of the mouth, till the morsel inside feels completely wet and fluid and easily makes its way to the stomach. Teach them to finish everything in the mouth before they go for the next bite. This is the long-term investment which will reap many health benefits.

3. Fresh seasonal fruits: Banana, mango, seetaphal, chikoo, jackfruit. The seasonal guava, pomegranate, grapes, apple, pear, peaches. The lesser-known and hyper local jamun, ber, white jaam, karvand, phalsa and the like — the wild and uncultivated fruits that are found in forests and may only be accessible one or two weeks of the year. Well, the child is growing and it's time to introduce her to all the goodness of the farms and forests of the region she lives in. Introduce kids to the concept of diversity of diets and seasonal eating by feeding them the fruits of the season but without making a noise about it.

The diversity of fruits has a lot to offer, from flavonoids, anthocyanins and anti-oxidants to nutrients and benefits still unknown to nutrition science. They make the gut resilient, prevent sicknesses related to change of season, work like a vaccination shot that prevents many diseases and risks in the future, and more importantly, keep tribal communities in business. A lot of kids these days have developed a natural aversion to fruits and i suspect it's because we are feeding them the kiwis, the apples and the tangerines that are available year-round, sourced from places across the globe, and naturally then going through long logistical chains and also not very eco-friendly methods of production. If your child is one of those, switch them to the local fruit, buy them from local markets and watch miracles happen. Also then, look at your child with a glint of grudging respect in your eyes; she was not fruit averse, only chemical averse.

How to feed: Again, mash or cut in small pieces as required, remove seeds if any and then feed. With jamun and stuff, once they are grown up, you can teach them how to eat from one side, remove the seed and then eat the other side. As they grow, teach them to wash the fruit on their own and eat. Take them to farms once a month or as often as you can, and let them watch how fruits grow on trees, ripen, mature and are taken down for humans to eat. How human beings share this food with bees, birds and other living beings. Kids learn more by watching and observing than by hearing, so keep the speech short and give them the time to stand and stare, even smell.

OVERFEEDING

At a shraadh function, a young mother sat next to me with her kid in her lap. As the hosts began serving rice on the banana leaf, she switched on her iPhone and let her son watch. Then rasam-rice, sambar-rice, dahi-rice, she fed the son everything that was served. i am forty, the son was four, max; he easily ate four times more than me, eyes glued to the screen, and four times faster than me. Just as i was about to wrap my banana leaf and get up, the son began to throw up — in the reverse order — first came dahi-rice, then sambar-rice, followed by rasam-rice. i was nauseous enough at the sight of his eating, now his puking was the real test. Well, i passed and managed to move without throwing up myself, but this urge to feed kids a lot and quickly needs to be nipped in the bud. Let them eat just one thing, but let them watch what they are eating and let them take their time. Because a sick baby is costliest in terms of time. And time is the only thing that human beings actually own or can call their own. So let's work at optimising the time on earth where they are at their supreme health and nothing else.

iii) Five to Eight Years

These are the years before puberty and the time to optimise calcium stores. This is officially when children begin to create an identity of their own. They begin to understand biases, gender differences, etc. They are also most likely to fall for food marketing at this age, as it's an impressionable age. And the impressions they begin to make now will live with them and influence their personality and well-being for a long time to come. And so, if you go by the Sanskrit subhashit, if until five years of age you must be lenient and indulgent with your children, then for ten years starting from five, you must not hesitate to discipline them. *Dasha varshani tadayat* goes the subhashit, literally meaning, beat for the next ten years, but in essence meaning no giving in to tantrums, teaching them where to draw the line and being disciplined with food and timings.

If you look at it from the bone mineral density (BMD) point of view, it makes perfect sense. They make huge gains in their BMD starting now, and this sets the pace for them to reach their peak BMD well into their thirties. If there is too much weight loss talk, diet discussions, food being broken down to carbs, protein, fat on the dinner table, i promise you they are going to get nowhere close to where their BMD should be. And that leads to poor physical performance, low vitamin D levels, and a difficult puberty, among many other things. So first let's make a commitment that you as parents will take the disciplined route and follow all the parent fundas listed out in Part 1 and ensure that the child is reaching peak bone mineral density by thirty-five and staying effortlessly healthy and happy.

Before we get going with food though, this is the age when you must start implementing the ninety minutes free play, per day, compulsorily. And you won't have any trouble doing it if you have access to open spaces within your complex, society or live near a public park. If you don't, try and create opportunities for this, and as i said earlier, even shift homes if needed. Then, within the household, start getting them involved in the kitchen. They can start setting curd, bringing food out, picking up their own plate. Taking their own tiffin out from the school bag, washing it and drying it. Watering plants with what is left in the water bottle, rinsing it and drying it. Making their own bed, tying their own shoelaces, putting all chappals back on the rack. But please, lead by example; if this is going to come as a lecture, it's not going to happen. And your status, richness, wealth will only increase if the child is more self-reliant, so bindaas have them move — don't make them suffer your wealth, please.

Alright, back to business now. **The top three foods for five–eight years**:

1. Makhan: White butter or cultured butter, as the US high-end stores like to call it, is essential for a child of this age group. For multiple reasons, but most importantly because it allows them to keep the mobility in their joints.

Your child may only be five or six, but you will notice that they are no longer able to put their toes in their mouth the way they used to when they were five months old. Part of it is the natural growth process, but if you leave it unattended, it will lead to poor bone density and the risk of osteoporosis at a later stage.

The makhan that i am referring to will need to be made at home, employing the traditional processes of using live bacteria culture so that it has all the goodness that it needs to have. A rich, essential fatty acid profile, storehouse of all fat soluble vitamins A, D, E, K and the magic of the Wulzen factor (a hormone-like substance which allows bones to get stronger). Together they keep the young body free of all diseases, adequate on vitamin D and make it super easy for the body to load up and gain on BMD. The child begins to look stronger and leaner. The vitamin K2 present in makhan is of great importance, because it ensures that the body gets the right signals to load up the calcium stores in the bones and teeth. Along with that, it works at keeping the insulin sensitive so that puberty is smooth and obesity is kept at bay. Research says that obesity under ten is linked to cancer risk at a later age. So don't worry about keeping them golu-molu; instead, let them grow strong and lean.

How to eat: First, involve them in making makhan — they love it. The front and back action with the wooden churner, the particles coming together to form an airy white mass that floats on water, and the light aroma of the fresh butter. Some of the naturally skinny people i have worked with often tell me how their grandma fed them dollops of white butter while churning it. Higher the bone density, lower the body fat — that's the connect here.

You can have the makhan with roti or bhakri, make a murukku or chaklis with it, have it as butter tea in the Himalayan regions of India, or have it with thalipeeth or chillas. The options are endless. If you are looking for inspiration, just look into your food heritage and #beinspired. You can even bake an occasional nankatai with it.

Also, makhan has almost zero levels of lactose, so don't worry if the kid is lactose intolerant, it is safe. And please don't confuse this with store-bought yellow butter; this is different and way better. Makhan or white butter also works at improving digestive processes and improves diversity of gut-friendly bacteria. For this, you will also have to follow the food heritage in totality and buy desi cow milk or milk from the local dairy, so that it hasn't gone through the processes of homogenisation and pasteurisation. As far as safety of milk goes, for centuries the native cultures of India, Middle East, Africa have known how to use fresh milk and ensure that it's safe to drink — boil it before using it.

MAKHAN AND VITAMIN A

Now that we use so much industrialised and packaged milk, we are losing out on the many advantages that milk products like makhan offer. Makhan, made traditionally, is rich in vitamin A, the one vitamin that looks after your immune system, teaching it to fight every disease without ever falling sick. The misinformation about cholesterol meant that traditional milk-drinking societies were put off makhan and ghee. Then the food industry offered low-fat butters and alternatives like margarine. Now that the ill-effects of the low-fat substitutes are known, they are offering to fortify rice with vitamin A in Africa and maybe our atta or biscuits. The point is that the food industry will keep turning us into profit-making entities and, one after another, we will lose out on our food heritage, and become sick societies that live longer with diseases. This can't be the future for our children — it needs to change with us, now.

2. Handful of peanuts: For many reasons — the vitamin B profile, the rich mineral content, the amino acids, basically everything that is needed to support the growing body. Not to mention the yummy taste. Plus, the fact that peanuts —

or any legume, dal or pulse — is great for our soil too. Soil, as you are aware, is a non-renewable resource. The future of our planet lies in good soil health, and when peanuts and other legumes are sowed, they enrich the soil with nitrogen, good bacteria and many other nutrients. Peanuts, or singdana as they are called, are considered amongst the world's healthiest foods. Their polyphenol content protects the heart better than red wine (red wine is not good — it just has good publicity); its fatty acid profile is better than olive oil (btw, producing olive oil to meet world demand has turned it into a highly polluting industry); and what's more, it even prevents the production of gall stones. Do a quick survey of people around you; you will know at least three people who have recently had a gall bladder removal surgery.

How to eat: Have a handful anytime during the day, turn it into a chutney that can be eaten with rotis, bhakris, parathas or dosas, mix it with jaggery and coconut and have it as a wholesome snack or a bus / after-school snack. Roasted peanuts have a slight nutritional advantage, that's why you will find that the most common way to eat them is roasted and salted or boiled and salted just when they are harvested. Chiki / gajak is good too. Do what you have to but get a handful a day.

In countries where there's high occurrences of peanut allergies, doctors are now suggesting two things: 1) Pregnant women should have peanuts every day so that their babies are born with stronger guts and the ability to digest peanuts. 2) For allergic children to get slow and tiny exposure to peanuts so they can build a tolerance for them. These countries aside, if your child is allergic or if you suspect he / she is, try putting a little peanut powder on your sabzis, koshimbirs and pachadis, a popular method of cooking in Maharashtra, Gujarat and in the south. And if you feel you just can't risk it, give a handful of chana instead. They come close to peanuts in their goodness. Can be eaten with jaggery too. Peanuts, chana, kurmura, roasted with salt, spices and curry leaves make for an easy, no-fuss, delicious evening snack also.

Please note: you can give them almonds, cashews, walnuts, etc., too, but not as a replacement for peanuts or chana.

3. **Papad**: Ha, ha. i bet you didn't see this coming, but here it is. The age where you introduce them to the good things in life. Where they learn to understand the common threads in our diverse cultures, and that irrespective of our region, religion, income, we all love our papad. Made from millets, lentils, potato, sabudana or your own unique preparation, by mixing ingredients with salt, spices and water (sometimes even flowed through banana stems), this is one of our artisan preparations. Is it healthy? Yes, very much so. i think you are done with people telling you what is healthy or unhealthy based on oil or salt or sugar. Kab, kaise, kitna, kis ke saath, kyun are some of the questions that you need to ask yourself.

i mean, at the end of the day, everything is about image and projection. Think about how many birthday parties you have attended, with kids wearing an apron and hat and rolling bloody pizzas as an activity and baking it. Uska fat and salt hum ko chaltay and papad ko tch tch? Come on, where is our self-esteem, our pride in our cuisine? Meanwhile, the Italians are tch tching you for eating pizza at a pizza chain. That's a rant for another day, but rethink positioning of food as rich and poor, please.

Alright, so the papad will obviously carry the nutrient profile of its base ingredients, be it the millet, lentil or the aloo. But there's more ways in which the papad has contributed to our culture. If you are around forty or even thirty-five, you must have made papad with more aplomb than your kid rolling pizza (you didn't even need the apron and the hat to feel important and it wasn't even a birthday) at your dadi's or nani's during summer. It brought the whole family together, boys and girls all employed in the kitchen tasks, running up and down the terrace to sun-dry this delicacy, and the endless stories that your grandma told you around it. Don't you want your kid to experience this?

And then the fact that when your favourite dal or sabzi was not made, you didn't throw a fuss, you just ate dahi, rice and papad. Or that when your mother had unexpected guests over, or a tough day, or you came back from a trip, you all just dug into khichdi and papad or kheechiya with some oil or ghee and masala sprinkled on it? And you needed nothing else: it tasted like heaven. The guests felt welcome and the host family not burdened by their arrival. A khichdi and papad kept families together, taught gender sensitivity and employed men in the kitchen without making a loud noise about equality or hashtags. There was no need for it — it was a way of life already. With the papad out of our lives, a lot of that togetherness, sensitivity, sharing is out of our lives. Children fuss about not having their favourite thing instead of digging into dal-rice with papad. The papad was also a lesson in adjustment and self-reliance, without meaning to be one.

How to eat: Kheechiya, deep-fried papad (always better than roasted, it's tastier and you end up eating less too), papad and dahi, and if you are a Sindhi, even sabzi and milkshake. The key to remember here is, fikar not, your child will never want a papad every day, but it makes for a good accompaniment when they don't fancy the sabzi at dinner or have friends over or during winter or a rainy day. And your child is sensible, so she will self-terminate the act of eating papad; it will also teach her rationing because papads made at home are not endless in supply and must last an entire year. So there you go: a lesson in resource management too.

Note: All of the above is applicable for pickles, too. Made from fruits, seeds, veggies and berries, this is another artisan speciality from the Indian kitchens. Other than adding spice to your meal, pickles also add the much needed vitamin K (a co-factor in vitamin D assimilation) and diverse friendly bacteria (thanks to the lacto-fermentation process the pickles go through) to our diet. Both the papad and the pickle are vulnerable delicacies that may soon be a lost art.

The other art that is dying along with them is the sense of proportion the Indian thali intrinsically followed: the millet or grains like rice at the centre, the dal, sabzi at the right and the pickle, papad or chutney to the left. You eat more of what's in the centre, a little less of what's on the right and the least of what's on the left. But when you eat it all together, you experience all the six tastes, the rasa of life. And that it's a perfectly balanced nutritious meal, is a bonus.

iv) Eight to Twelve Years

Everything that you did from five to eight will begin to show its effects now and will ensure that you hit a smooth ride into puberty. While some of you may hit puberty by twelve, some of you may reach it by fifteen, and some even later. Each one of us is on our own unique growth curve, one that is determined by genes, physical activity, stress levels, food pattern, pollution levels and — very importantly — sleep. So don't be in a rush to hit puberty; know that it is a natural occurrence which will happen in its own sweet time. Now, of course, feel free to ask your parents and school counsellors questions, and ensure that they are answered in a way that you understand.

It breaks my heart to say this, but some girls will drop out from regular playing at this age itself. If you are one of those girls, come on, buck up. You have to play at least till you turn twenty-three so that you can optimise growth and fitness, and you are not even half of that age yet. And don't worry about company — if no one else is playing, you still keep up with it. Girls have this important job of doing their own thing, whether or not the others are following. You have to live your own life on your own terms. Same with boys; don't trade play time with video games (especially the PUBG, Fortnite types) or staring at a screen with another group of boys.

This is traditionally the time to get children to either practice five suryanamaskars every day, enrol in a classical art — music, dance, instrument anything at all you fancy (at least once a week) — or start learning a martial art. You can do all three, but you should at least commit to doing two of the above. The suryanamaskars, especially — they keep the core strong and joints mobile, and ensure that kids have a smooth ride hormonally. So their puberty is one that doesn't lead to confusion or withdrawal but is one that they are able to take in their stride.

And with this, the other important thing to do is to say no to sleep-overs. Sleep is closely linked to hormonal health, and your little girl or boy staying up all night, loading up on cakes and chocolates, who knows even caffeine, lounging on the bed or sofa and watching the screen, is what hormonal disasters are made of. So no, don't out-do the classmate who hosted the sleepover at a 5-star; just don't play that game. And if you really must, then no more than two sleepovers in a year. Come on, as a parent it's your job to say no, so say it. Do a little advocacy in the PTA or the mommy WhatsApp group or take a pic of this para and post it there. Hopefully, the other parents will also buy and read the full book: it will solve your troubles and make me more royalties; win-win. The child wins too, hurray.

PERIOD

We all worry that girls are hitting puberty earlier these days, sometimes as young as eight or ten. Well, i seriously want every girl to get her period only by fourteen, at least post twelve, and same with boys — hit puberty after twelve. The silver lining is that parents today are more open to talking about periods, and it's not some state secret that everyone knows but no one talks about. Having said that, don't stress out your little girl over it. And when the period comes, give it till she is fifteen to get regular; don't pump her with hormones to get a period every month at ten or twelve. It's natural for the period cycle to take three to five years to set itself in a routine. In the meanwhile, give her good food, ask her to maintain good sleep habits and ensure that she has free play of ninety minutes per day, in addition to at least two of the activities listed above. Sixty minutes is the bare minimum for free play — it's just too little, it ends even before they begin to get into the groove of getting anywhere close to their maximal power, strength or stamina, so push for ninety. Let them bunk a class or even school, but not play time.

Also, even if you have just a boy and no girl, do the period talk. Let him grow up knowing about life as it is and not like some alien who's indifferent to the physiology of the other half of the population.

So, back to food business — **top three foods for eight–twelve**:

1. Sherbets: Homemade, of course. You can make all kinds, nimbu being the easiest of them all. Let me tell you Alia Bhatt's favourite nimbu sherbet recipe: nimbu, sugar, a little grated adrak, kalanamak, one or two strands of kesar, a freshly crushed pepper. Ah! You have a natural, vitamin and electrolyte-rich drink that can pound any sports drink to the ground with its looks, taste and beverage hydration index. It cools your body down, allows for your skin to clear up and makes for a great meal during or post play. Slurp, slurp.

You can make all kind of sherbets — mogra, khus, kokum, amla, bel — the key is to make it yourself, then it tastes sweeter. Even better is to become the official sherbet person of the family and friend circle; you will literally have people eating, oops, drinking out of your hands. Sherbets make for a good digestive, allow the core body temperature to cool down and most ingredients in regional Indian sherbets even allow for better hormonal balance.

Needless to say, avoid packaged juices, readymade mixes like flavoured drinks, and colas and caffeinated drinks (sherbets from small women's cooperatives are ok, though). According to Ayurveda, the tongue can taste six different tastes: sweet, sour, salty, bitter, pungent, astringent. Indian sherbets were meant to stoke the appetite and sensitise the tongue to experience all the six tastes. This is the time when the appetite surges and a tongue that is trained to gather all tastes, gathers the most benefits from the food that is eaten. It is important that parents remind children to eat slowly at this age, instead of fussing over the quantities or experimenting with portions. The slower they eat, the sharper the feedback from the tongue, the better they learn to chew and terminate eating at the right point. Typically, this will be the age group where your grandma reminded you to not count how much you ate but to eat just as much as you need.

How to drink: As a mid-meal or during or post a game. You can even make yourself a fresh fruit milkshake if you fancy that instead of a sherbet or if you are hungrier for more than a sherbet. Take the pulp out fresh, mix it in milk and churn it with the ravi (wooden churner) instead of a blender where you could lose out on the nutrients from the fruit. Or you could even make yourself a nicely beaten lassi with some kesar and sugar or just by itself or with salt; play with it based on how you feel. Let your creative juices flow, chef.

A MEMORY

Memories are a wonderful thing and they are often made of taste and smell of food. One of my favourite ones is connected to nimbu sherbet. i was ten and on a summer vacation to Chiplun in Konkan with my grandfather, Appa. My playmate was my maasi, Pallavi, who was just a year older than me. When you have a large family, sometimes your cousins are years younger than you, and uncles and aunts are your age. Anyway, we were bored and seeking some adventure. Climb to the top of the hill in kaju cha adva, said Appa. It was a little forest by the house. So Pallavi and i made nimbu sherbet — we squeezed the lemons in our water bags (that's what you had in the 1980s), added sugar and salt, and shook it till our deltoids hurt, to mix it properly. Appa tasted it and told us that we were good to go. Up we went to the little forest and trudged all the way to the top of the hill. Once on top, we opened our water bags and drank. Amrit; i tasted amrit on that day. It was so good that i almost gave up drinking nimbu sherbet after that day because i didn't want to spoil the memory of that taste.

2. Legumes / pulses: A serving a day. Should be soaked overnight, preferably allowed to sprout, and then cooked well by adding a pinch of sendha namak. Many reasons, but these will give the hormones the stability they require, the muscles the strength they need and the bones the density they require. India has a large variety to choose from — 65,000 different types of pulses, can you beat that? And you know the hierarchy, right? The best farm produce is turned into usal or sundals, the second-best to dals, the third best to wadis or papads, and the last grade made into a cake for cattle. Zero wastage has been the Indian farmer's moola mantra; smart, na.

So you would need to diversify and go beyond just the chana, rajma, chickpea, masur, matki, moong, etc. My recommendation is surely kulith (horsegram); get that on your weekly rotation menu and then look around for more delicacies of your region — like the navrangi dal of Garhwal. These make for a very good source of fibre too, and can be cooked in multiple ways.

How to eat: Obviously as accompaniments to rice, rotis or bhakris. Also as chillas and ghavans, eaten with dahi or chutney — makes for an excellent, wholesome, delicious and nutritious snack. The kulith is also turned into a soupy preparation and with a dollop of makhan or ghee will help you prevent kidney stones, keep skin supple and fight that flu for you. It could make for a great late-night meal if you are up studying (which i hope you are not) or would make for a wholesome dinner on a day you want something light for your system. If you play intense, serious sports, like looking to crack district / state level, repeat the kulith every two to three days as a dal to go with rice, especially for dinner. Other ways of eating legumes and lentils are sundals, which make for a great snack or even for a rushed breakfast.

Mamai had this routine where, once every week, she made me and my sister and her two biological granddaughters (all four of us and she, we were a gang) a really special dish called kalan. Actually we made special things for our gang all the time, but this was our favourite. We would save up sour dahi for this, and then when no one else was around, we would mix the really sour dahi or chaas into kulith dal and turn it into kalan. A special, Konkani dish that optimises the B12 assimilation and puts sour dahi to use (instead of wasting it), turning into a delicacy by mixing it with a nutrient-rich dal.

Legumes and lentils are diverse in their nutrient profile, preparations and taste, so make the most of it. Laddoos, barfis and even halwas are made with dals in India. While the laddoo and barfi are similar, just differently moulded, they make for a good snack, or can be had with milk as a breakfast meal too. Halwas are typical of many festivals, can speed up recovery from a bout of illness and even work as a dessert post lunch on special occasions.

3. Aliv or garden cress seeds: It's one of the ten foods that i wrote about in my book *Indian Super Foods*; it even makes it to my list of recommendations in *Pregnancy Notes;* and now it's here too, as the super food for the eight to twelve bracket. Well, it's the chota bomb with bada energy. Rich in iron and folic acid, this is exactly what you need to push up your haemoglobin stores, nurture your thyroid gland and speed up recovery after long play sessions. These are tiny seeds, the size of til, but blood red in colour. They have a nice, unique taste of their own and having a teaspoon every day will even give your skin, hair and nail health a boost. Surely a must-have if you have a history of low haemoglobin levels, are anaemic or have anyone in the family with BP or IBS issues. The aliv will help you prevent those in the future too.

How to eat: My favourite is an aliv laddoo. Made with aliv seeds, ghee, coconut and jaggery, it's a great and fulfilling mid meal, just perfect for the small break at school. It immediately lifts you out of boredom and lethargy and renews you with a fresh lease of life. It's perfect to prevent mood swings and irritability too. You can even add a teaspoon to your nariyal pani or a cup of milk and have it. They can be added to khakharas, theplas and parathas, or you could simply chew on them, like saunf, post a meal. Happy chewing.

v) Twelve to Fifteen Years

The world is a beautiful place, but being a teenager is a rough ride, especially in these times. When i see some mommies of teenagers and the duck face they make when taking a selfie, i am unable to tell who the teen is. Same with some daddies who go to Goa and Thailand with their 'boys', who are other forty-year-olds. There really is something called as age-appropriate behaviour, and it's high time we learn that so that we make life a little easier for our teens. Teenage is basically a rough ride because we are on the journey to discover our footing, our place in this world. To figure that the world is like a cup of tea, it becomes what you make of it and that it gets better with time. The more you are able to tell who you really are versus who you are being made out to be based on what you wear, eat and speak, the more you begin to discover your real self. And once you get that glimpse of who you really are, you are no longer tempted to be anything other than yourself, and that is the key to unending health, joy and happiness. Eating right makes that journey easier; as i said earlier, anna is the journey to ananda. But in 2018, the generation that has lived before you has ushered you into a journey of climate change.

As you get older, the more you will begin to understand the health and economic downsides of climate change. You have probably received a shot for every communicable disease out there, maybe a dozen so far, but what is really going to get us is climate change. The vector-borne diseases that come with it (the latest one is where the platelet count crashes, but it's not dengue or any other known condition), the change in gut-friendly bacteria, allergies and intolerances, and finally the NCDs — top five being diabetes, heart disease, cardio pulmonary diseases, cancer and mental health issues. Well, with your daily choices though, you can find a footing of your own, review all that is being sold to you and figure out how to eat and live in a climate-resilient manner.

Since you are grown-ups, i will keep my instruction short for you. You already know what to do and what to avoid, so here goes — **top three foods for twelve–fifteen**:

1. Dal-rice-sabzi-ghee for dinner: The coolest kids are the ones who have the simplest dinners. This combination of rice, dal and ghee gives you a complete amino acid profile and gives a stimuli for your body to drive up the growth spurt. It is also the easiest grain to digest and ensures you get a good night's sleep, so essential at this age. You can even have a roti or bhakri with dal and sabzi. You can also add a pickle or a papad to your dinner. And if you have home-set curd, you can have that for dinner as well. The dal can be replaced regularly with sprouted and cooked legumes or you can have them at some other point in the day, either for lunch or as a chilla for an evening snack. Sabzi should be seasonal and local, and the one that is being made for the rest of the household — you know that by now.

How to eat: Without gadgets, without a fuss, without fear, and early in the night. *Aath chya aat bhaat, pot sapat,* goes a line in Marathi. It means that if you want a flat stomach, you must finish dinner with rice before 8 p.m. Rice is also one of the foods that Kareena Kapoor ate to ensure that she had a flat stomach for the promotions of *Veere di Wedding*. It puts you in a good mood and high-energy levels through the day, so that you may quickly recover from boring classes and tiring sports practice. It allows you to be the best version of yourself. Make sure that the rice is local, is hand-pounded or single polished, and not brown.

If you are bored of regular rice, you can have a khichdi, pulao or biryani instead, but it's important to keep your dinners simple. It reassures your body of a timely supply of nutrients and allows it to prioritise the most important metabolic function of growth and repair over anything else. In turn, it keeps you smart, both physically and mentally, and allows you to overcome the daily challenges of teenage life.

2. Cashews and raisins: You may not be aware, but cashews are a good source of minerals, iron especially and even magnesium, which help prevent bodily aches, pains and cramps. It got a bad rep for being high in cholesterol — that's typical nutritionism playing itself out; in fact, it has zero mg of cholesterol. And in any case, cholesterol is a much-needed anti-oxidant in the body, so no one should be avoiding it or taking meds to lower it. Instead, we should be taking daily steps to lower our misinformation.

Raisins are also much-loved and the perfect answer to the sweet cravings that you may have every once in a while. Perfectly natural and rich in iron, B6 and potassium, they are nature's cure for bloating, acidity and migraines / headaches. Do ensure that you get a daily dose of both. Especially needed if you get cramps during periods, have knee pain or a back that hurts and gets categorised as growing pains, or have frequent headaches or feel burnt-out by school stress.

How to eat: As a snack mid-morning or on the way back from school; it could also be a much-needed energy booster during long study hours and will leave you fresher and more awake than a cup of coffee or those caffeinated energy drinks. You can even add these to your shrikhand or halwa on special occasions. This is really quite the energy bomb that doesn't leave you with a slump later.

SUGAR TAX

While on coffee and caffeinated drinks and colas — these are pure poison for a growing body (leading to obesity and other NCDs), for your local economy and the globe's ecology at large. Other than the marketing and promotion, there is nothing else that is good about them. Enjoy their ads and don't touch the products. These are often the official sponsors of major cricket tournaments in our country and big sporting events, even Olympics, at a global scale. The very food companies that commit ecological theft by draining out ground water from the earth's resources, use celebs and packaging to position their junk as aspirational and sponsor sports tournaments in the hope that all the sporting greatness will deflect attention from the real damage that they cause to health and ecology. Sadly, for all of us, their techniques worked just fine — until recently.

It was a group of health campaigners from Mexico who really led the battle against cola companies, calling them out for the large amounts of poor quality sugar (HCFS or corn syrup), caffeine and other additives that they add to their products. Eventually, it led to many countries having a sugar tax that these food companies fought tooth and nail against, but finally relented to pay. The tax is very small and in no way compensates for the damage they have caused and continue to cause, but it's a step in the right direction.

i actually have a problem with it being called 'sugar tax', because then that puts even things like raisins and fresh fruit in the grey area. These have sugar too, but it's natural; there's a big difference. We should be calling it 'junk food tax' for the numerous chemicals, the plastic packaging and the addiction they cause. Only then will it be something worthwhile. Otherwise it will just be about one aspect or one nutrient: you lower or remove that and your junk can appear as healthy. In-our-face examples are baked chips, sugar-free colas, packaged fruit juices, etc.

3. **Chutneys every day**: This young, adolescent age is a stepping stone towards adulthood. And what we do know is that, other than obesity and malnutrition deaths, the other burden that we face is of hidden hunger. There are approximately two billion micronutrient-deficient people in the world. These are people with low levels of haemoglobin, vitamin D, vitamin B12 and many other

micronutrients, and these deficiencies — or hidden hunger as it is called — prevents you from experiencing human life to its fullest. It keeps you in the loop of having frequent illnesses, and increases your risk to obesity and NCDs too. The thing to remember here is that if you are low on even one micronutrient, it means that you are low on many others too.

Going back to traditional methods of eating is a guaranteed way of ensuring that your body receives all the micronutrients that are required. It allows your body and brain to grow optimally and function at its best. Traditionally, our food heritage was full of chutneys that we made from leaves, seeds and even roots and barks. We are fast losing those to the ketchups and hot sauces of the world. Chutneys made from curry patta, alshi (flaxseed), coconut, dals, even bhang, and eaten with rotis, sometimes even mixed with rice or as an accompaniment to khakra, paratha, idli, etc., meant that the body received its dose of essential fatty acids, micro minerals, vitamins and other phytonutrients. In Udupi, they even have the tradition of mixing these chutneys into chaas. According to the season, they make it either with hibiscus flower or other leaves; very interestingly, one is called vitamin soppu because it has all the nutrients out there.

How to eat: Chutneys are a great way to spice up life and make interesting out of boring. They can give your regular breakfast, lunch and dinner good company. Chew your grandmom's head and find out the ones that are rarely used now — they will most likely be made out of seeds and leaves. These are good to keep pimples at bay too, as they often work at optimising blood sugar and improving the functioning of insulin. Such a tasty way to stay thin. These are even better than your peanut or almond butter on bread. You could make a sandwich using these and makhan, and if you don't like makhan then just the chutney mixed in groundnut or mustard oil, and use it like a yum spread on bhakri or bread.

Important note: Eating out

'Bachhe aate hai toh kya khate hai?' i asked a popular chef in a Landour restaurant which sees a steady stream of students from Dehradun and Mussourie. 'Pizza, pasta, burger, sandwich,' he replied without wasting a moment. 'Also potato wedges, pancakes, waffles. Bachho ko taste se koi matlab nahi hota.' 'Matlab?' i prodded. 'Taste kaisa bhi ho, appearance acha hona chahiye,' he explained. Well, he's not completely off the mark; teenage is that kind of age where the cover is more important than content. Part of it is just age, part of it is the fact that desi food in restaurants is totally blah, no matter how posh the restaurant.

If you are a committed chef, you must make the effort to showcase local in a good light and the young ones will opt for that over the regular junk stuff, says my gut. And if you are one of the young ones, then here, listen to my observation. Every time i see you kids sitting in restaurants and eating, clicking selfies, laughing in a natural rhythm, i always feel a tinge of guilt that we adults have failed you in many ways. There should have been greener spaces for you to meet; wide open, where birds fly and flowers blossom. Where you could come with a picnic basket from home and have a whale of a time. Run, shout, eat, laugh, all to your heart's content.

Now when i see you lounging in restaurants — sloppy backs, podgy stomachs, junk on plate — i know my generation created this for you. All of us forty-somethings, we were fitter than you are at your age, mostly because we hardly ever ate out, a couple of times a year, max. We had more open spaces, but we traded those for concrete buildings. We expected to make more wealth; instead, we lost it because health is the only wealth that counts, rest is just numbers. But every time i interact with you guys in schools or when you come with your parents on my retreats, i know that you will change the world, correct the mistakes of my generation. That fire in your stomach, may it burn bright and may it be fed all the local, seasonal food that belongs to your heritage. Tathastu.

Part 2b — Occasion-Wise

1) School days

There was a time when schools would be open for just about six hours. i went to one such school, Seth Chunilal Damordas Barfiwala High School; don't laugh, it's a real school. The society where i lived and the school shared a boundary wall, so i ran to and back from school without getting out of breath, not because of my fitness but because it was next door.

Nowadays, of course, schools have turned into a 7.30 / 8 a.m. to 3.30 / 4 p.m. affair; it's like the whole day is just gone, whoosh. And if that coveted school is far off, then the kid is just in the bus / car, and much more importantly, in traffic, forever. They wake up at some unrealistic hour to make it on time, often missing out on the very important early morning sleep, which is critical for growth. They have very little time left for free play or to genuinely pursue a hobby or an interest, and then almost all meals are outside; even if they take food from home, it's still not fresh. So max they have three meals at home, and very often even those are rushed, so no time to sit and eat, forget sit and stare. It's like being rushed through the phase of childhood without the luxury of time.

My sister is from IIM-A, and along with her husband who is an IIT-B and IIM-A specimen, she runs the most sought-after school in Surat: Fountainhead School. Rashmi Bansal also had a chapter on them in her first book. They are a couple driven by their passion for education, change and an equitable society, but also thoda hi-fi types, you get the drift. Like when i signed up for a women entrepreneur three-month course from a local Mumbai college, my sister told me — you are doing a C-grade course from a B-grade university. 'Chalega mere ko,' i told her, 'i am a Z grade person.' But basically, they are this smart couple; my bro-in-law was even head of campus recruitments in IIM-A, but opted out of every interview. This was way back in 2003; it made news and my sis took a job for a while to fund her and her bf's dream of the perfect school. They wanted to see their vision turn into reality at all costs and they did. But you ask my sister also, and she will say that the best school is the one which is next to your house. So that's her opinion, which i value very much. A school doesn't really matter, she told me, homes do. If you have the right environment at home, the child will succeed; baaki everything, this board, that board, everything is overrated.

So take my sister's free advice; unlike me, she is not a woman of many words, but when she does open her mouth, she has some pearls of wisdom, like this one — schools and boards are overrated.

Alright, the topic of what type of school is good for your kids is too tricky to cover in this book, so i will get back to what we can cover: **Food planning for a school day** to ensure that our kids are nourished well enough to enjoy their childhood, fight infections and overcome irritations that come their way.

Meal One — Before leaving for school

- Glass of plain water (kept overnight in a silver or kansa jar) + fresh local fruit or banana + some nuts and / or dry fruits and / or milk.
- Mix one nut and dry fruit. Cashew - raisin / Date – walnut / Dry dates – almonds / or a handful of mixed nuts (anything of their choice). If having badam, soak them overnight and ask the child to peel the skin before eating.
- Necessary to have at home, not in car, bus, etc.
- Sit and eat; last bite as you walk out of the door is ok, at the most.

Meal Two — Breakfast or mid-morning break at school.

- Hot homemade nashta — poha / upma / idli / dosa / paratha / idli / thukpa — anything belonging to your region and of your choice.
- Packed, but not in a plastic dabba, tissue, foil, etc.; instead, use malmal cloth or a handkerchief. Go green!

Meal Three — Lunch at school

- Roti-sabzi-dahi / dahi-rice-sabzi / usal or legumes with roti / any of the Meal Two options.
- Change millet as per season.
- Use ghee and makhan liberally.
- Don't forget chutneys or homemade achaar.

Meal Four — Typically at the end of school hours

This is also when they embark on the big ride back. Most fights, bullying will happen at this time, because they are already running low on sugar and can be hangry, cranky, irritable by this time.

- A glass of water, preferably from school, just to build gut resilience or from your own bottle.
- And a nice hydrating snack — banana, homemade laddoo, rajgeera chiki, cashews and raisins, homemade shrikhand, chivda, roti roll with jaggery and ghee.
- Other options — lassi or chaas or kokum / nimbu sherbet.

Meal Five — Mostly at home, wholesome and fresh

Go by what time they return and how hungry they are feeling. Options are:

- A legume or a millet prep — ragi satva or porridge or kheechiya or dosa or pulses / legume prep like sundal, chilla, etc., with dahi or white butter or ghee or meat, veggies and roti roll.
- Even a laddoo like aliv, or a mixture of coconut +

jaggery + peanuts, or chivda + dahi, or fresh fruit milkshake, etc.

- Banana with milk, sugar and roti (called shikran poli, a typical Maharashtrian, no-fuss meal).
- Sugarcane juice and kulith (i love the sound of this — it was a traditional meal in many parts of India till recently).
- Mango or banana or jackfruit and roti (the three fruits that are eaten with a meal, as per food heritage).
- Homemade chundos or chutneys with rotis or bhakris or rotlas.
- Or even poha or upma.

Meal Six — Dinner

- Anything rice based — pulao, khichdi, dal and rice. Can do roti-sabzi, roti-dal also if rice is not local to you.
- An example: waran bhaat with limbu, tup, meeth (rice and dal with lemon, salt and ghee, a typical Maharashtrian dish and Rohit Sharma's favourite, i am told).

Meal Seven — Before going to bed (if hungry)

- Milk, either plain or with gulkand or chyawanprash (depending on the season).

Points to remember:

- Do not enforce quantities or force them to have everything as per this plan — this is only for your reference. You have to fine tune it to the real school day. And according to number of classes post school, sports, etc., on that day.

- Based on the length of the day, you may need all of the above, or a couple less or a couple more meals.
- Play around with all the options listed, add more that fit the local – seasonal – food heritage formula.
- Expect them to be differently hungry on different days.
- Encourage them to: sit down for the meal; drink a glass of water before eating; serve only as per need; chew slowly; and sip on water during and post the meal as needed.
- Ideally, plan the menu a week in advance with the child's help. Engage them in grocery shopping, kitchen work, packing and cleaning the school dabba for better compliance to the meal plan and to encourage them to eat responsibly.
- No biscuits, packaged juices, cereals, jams, dips, chips, chocolates, colas, etc., on a daily basis.

BIRTHDAYS IN SCHOOL

Most schools have now adopted a no celebrating birthday in school, no chocolate, cake, etc., policy.

> Good on you, but let the kid celebrate also ya, a bit. Birthdays are a good time to emphasise on growing up and being responsible. It's a good time to showcase delicacies that are unique to your region, community, family, and get everyone to bite into the various influences on your cuisine. Don't let this opportunity pass, by coming up with some half-baked ideas like no cakes, only cupcakes. How is that resolving anything at all? But 'only homemade delicacy' policy will. It will improve the diet diversity of all school kids, help them understand each other better, produce no wastage or garbage and can be turned into something unique that everyone looks forward to. This exercise is a hundred times more useful than pasting pictures and making a family tree. Once it's connected to food, 'where i come from' is much more real for a kid.

Special note: Exams

Here are some food strategies that will equip you mentally and physically to cope with the challenges of exams:

i. A month before exams
   - Keep yourself hydrated by having traditional drinks like coconut water, buttermilk, kokum sherbet, panna, etc.

- Have a wholesome meal between 4 and 6 p.m., the time you are most likely to feel fatigued. Some options are: cheese sandwich, chapatti with ghee and sugar or jaggery, chivda and dahi, a fresh fruit milkshake.
- If you are studying late in the night, you can have dry fruits, nuts, a milkshake or options mentioned above.

ii. A day prior to the exam
- No instant noodles, chocolates, cupcakes.
- Ensure that you spare at least sixty minutes to play / exercise.
- Take a power nap during the day; it will help you retain what you study.
- Include dahi in your meals; it will help with any exam stress-related indigestion issues.
- Strictly no energy or caffeinated drinks — they come in the way of brain function and performance.

iii. On the exam day
- Have a fresh, homemade breakfast.
- Follow the ritual of having dahi cheeni or fresh fruit before exams.
- Carry some nimbu pani or kokum sherbet in a small bottle and sip it during the exam.
- Immediately after the paper, either have a fresh fruit like banana or a wholesome meal like poha, homemade laddoo, ghee-jaggery-roti, etc.

2) Holidays

These are the best days of your life. As children, you should ideally experience these four types of holidays every year:

i. Go and stay at the home of a relative — grandparents, bua, mama, masi, chacha, tau, etc. — at least a couple of nights without parents.

ii. Stay in your own home without the routine of school and classes.

iii. Relatives or friends at your home.

iv. Holiday within India — possible at all budgets and hopefully involving some trekking, skiing, beach, deserts, forests, safaris, farms, forts, etc.

Strictly optional, holiday v — a holiday abroad. But please, no Dubai and Singapore (after fifteen is fine, but surely not before five; you can't possibly teach them that in malls, shopping and theme parks lies the good life). These days, what i think is strictly optional is all that kids seem to be doing, because of their parents. Parents to blame, always.

Ok, let me tell you why all these kinds of holidays are important. They are important because it means children get exposed to different water, foods and living conditions. Water here is most important; it influences and changes the food, language, culture and, of course, people. Besides, people who have drunk all kinds of water build a resilient gut, an adaptable mind and an undeterred focus. *Barah gaav cha paani pyayliye ti*, is often said to describe a woman who's seen it all (coz she had water from twelve different villages) and won't get bogged down by small troubles (little grudgingly though, but you get the point).

Why these holidays?

Holiday 1: Allows them to intrinsically understand how to behave like a good guest; helps them climb down from a sense of entitlement and yet be indulged and loved by the family. They also begin to get a sense of how home routines, kitchens and food habits impact the health and fitness of the members of the family. Without you saying much, they learn valuable life lessons about conducting themselves responsibly, adjusting palates and meal timings and bonding over differences. This is the stuff that prepares them for life, not the chocolate buffet on the cruise. And like i said earlier, don't call and inform the hosts what the kid likes or dislikes. Once they are outside their home, most times, they are happy to eat everything without making a fuss. And if something really is a problem, they will even learn to find the words to voice it. So all good.

Holiday 2: Enables them to tell the difference between real life and a break. This is the time they can use to play extra, sleep extra, eat extra and revel in it all. To have friends over longer, maybe also to play longer indoor games. Basically, be at home and chill. This is your one chance to get the kid to observe all that goes into running an efficient home. And over a period of time, they will begin to value all the background things that keep churning so that their school, classes, etc., happen without any disturbance. This is also a good time to involve them in the kitchen: make a laddoo, shrikhand, pickle together, or maybe go shopping for the kitchen. Or simply get them to clean up both the kitchen and their own wardrobes.

Holiday 3: Is very important; it's your chance to share and truly show that you care. These are the holidays where the child learns to put herself second and the guest first. They learn the fine balance between give and take and understand what behaviour from a guest can be burdensome and what is an absolute pleasure, and therefore figure out how they should behave the next time someone plays host to them. The first and third type of holidays are almost disappearing from our modern lives and getting fast replaced by playdates. A playdate ends before you truly learn to adjust with the friend or cousin, so it's only more consumption and entertainment. Holidays are an opportunity to learn how to stick it out through all kinds of situations, what to let go of, what to hold on to, so that we create the best time for ourselves and everyone around.

THE LITTLE THINGS

One of my grandaunts was notorious for making really small portions of sabzis. She would make usal-bhakris-rice-dahi, all according to the number of people, but the sabzi was exactly one katori. And then because the sabzi was so little, everyone would either have very little of it or nothing at all. Post that she would declare that, though the whole family teases her about her sabzi portions, the fact was that whatever little she makes also gets left over. 'None of you eat bhaji,' she said to me, but it was meant for my granduncle. 'If you make more, maybe we will eat more,' i said on his behalf, and my cousins high-fived me. 'Ah! Pearls of the same string,' she said about all of us, my granduncle and all the grandkids of his various brothers. My granduncle winked at us, and one of my cousins said, 'Come on, don't feel bad, this was just a suggestion.' 'Well, i have a suggestion for all of you,' she said. 'Keep your mouth shut while eating and don't feel the compulsion to use the tongue just because you have one.' Life lessons over bhendi sabzi.

Holiday 4: Allows them to dip into culture, history, geography and understand how they influence the locals, the food, the environment at large. They are also able to see how the same junk food makes an appearance whether it's a beach, mountain, or even Ganga ghat, and how its packaging pollutes, whether it's a lake, a valley or a city. So they experience food distribution and marketing of junk food or poor positioning of local, healthy food outside of a classroom and textbook. This learning is more valuable than the ability to read food labels, which hardly tells you anything about how industry influence, policymaking, etc., affects public health at large. It's not about healthy choices, it's about healthy policies that put people first and not profits. And no, you don't have to say all this to them, they will figure this out by themselves, keen observers that they are. And over a period of time, they will make sense of all that they saw and bring about a healthy environment for themselves.

Holiday 5: i have a theory: the more you feed your children pasta, etc., at home, the more likely you are to carry thepla / khakra when you are travelling abroad. The thing, though, is that when you are out there, let them absorb the environment around them. They will even be able to figure out why there is bad news around carbs or sugar, because everything from muffins to breakfast cereal to breads to dessert post dinner is how they consume sugar and carbs, not like us at home with our fresh preparations. How expensive hotels or even business class travel offer you only packaged juices, and how people consume more of that than fresh fruit. How stuff like quinoa is available across the world in Paris, Budapest, London, New York, Miami, Sydney, etc., when it is actually non-native to each one of these places. An exposure like this, too, can save them from diet fads later, but only if you have managed to clean up the food environment at home. They may also be able to see how much better behaved you are to staff outside as compared to back home ;-).

Coming to food, here is a suggested **holiday eating plan**:

Meal One: Nuts or fruit (if the gap between waking up and eating is less than twenty to forty minutes).

Meal Two: Breakfast — anything homemade or a local delicacy or peanut butter-toast or egg if travelling abroad.

Meal Three: Sherbets — kids could make these themselves (lemonade, etc., if abroad).

Meal Four: Lunch — dahi-rice / roti-sabzi / pasta or pizza (based on where you are travelling) — but something local and seasonal.

Meal Five: Nuts or homemade laddoo or pieces of pickle or papad that you are making or chiki or a fresh fruit.

Meal Six: Something nice and chatpata that is homemade — kachori, samosa or a local chaat or chivda or chakli / murukku or mathri or suhali (stuff that is made at home and stays fresh for about a week or two). A smoothie or the best pastry money can buy (when travelling).

Meal Seven: Dinner — dal-chawal or versions of rice, beans or cottage cheese or tofu with veggies in any cuisine, regional or international, depending on your travel, or very simply khichdi and papad or kadhi or dahi. Or the occasional pav bhaji.

Meal Eight: Gulkand milk or haldi milk (if they are up till late and want to have something).

Holidays are a stimulating environment for kids — expect their appetite to increase and ensure that good food is accessible at all times. Encourage them to eat slowly though, and only that much so they can eat the next meal in the next two to three hours. If they have stuffed themselves and are later feeling uncomfortable, remind them to eat aaraam se and not all at once. A stuffed or a hungry kid is cranky and it's a loop — they will eat so much that they are not hungry for hours, then get so hungry that when they eat there is no stopping them. Help them establish four meal timings out of the eight listed. And as long they stick to those, they will have a good time. (If they are munching in between, allow that.) In school they eat on time because of a set routine, so holidays are a time for them to learn how to stay within a framework even when they don't really have to stick to a schedule.

Important notes

1. *Meal ideas for long flights*

i. Firstly, as a parent, please don't drink alcohol on the

flight. Actually, parenthood means saying no to every free drink out there. Fly and land in your senses, please. And if you feel that you are very much in your senses post a drink or two, you are exactly the reason why this point comes first.

ii. Always carry rice, ghee and metkut — this is a great, no fuss meal to have on flights. Will keep them full, less likely to opt for the junk and is light on the stomach. Please do this on short haul, domestic flights too.

iii. Encourage children to drink water; carry their own water bottle for this and there must be at least one sussu every three / three-and-a-half hours, unless of course they are sleeping.

iv. Chiki or laddoo are good ideas too, and help keep the chocolates at bay.

v. Before boarding the flight, especially if it's a long one or ones where only junk food is served, discuss what is that one thing they would like to have. Allow them to have that one thing, but tell them to divide it in four equal parts and eat only one part. This is only if you are currently weaning them off junk food, because then it's tough to get them to go from 100 to zero overnight, but you can always regulate. The fact is that even as flights dehydrate and disturb the digestion system, junk food only adds to that problem (even if it's free, and even if it's in first class, ok?).

vi. Airport food is slightly better than flight food, but

please don't eat chaat, pav bhaji, burgers and pizzas or even salads from chains. Actually point 6 cancel, just carry food from home — something like rice, banana, sandwich, depending on the length of the flight.

JUNK FOOD ON FLIGHTS

There's a saying in Afrikaans and Konkani: if you are not hungry for rice, you are not hungry. Ok, there isn't any such saying, but that is what this is all about. Every domestic flight you fly, especially the type where you buy meals on board, look at the amount of junk kids consume. So if it's holiday season and you are flying, the aircraft is smelling of MSG, the kids are patiently waiting for two to eight minutes for the boiled water to cook their poison, and the parents seem to give two hoots about killing their children, softly. Sorry, that's how i see it. The cartoon characters on the packaging, the ads during IPL, the experience of buying it, feeling all glam about it, is bound to tempt the child. Your job is to say no. Your job is to allow the child the freedom to throw a tantrum, cry, scream, kick the front seat (hold the leg in that case and say no, you can't do that; you can cry, though).

Let the whole aircraft look at you contemptuously, hold on to your composure and protect the poor kid. The ad council may not have the ethics to stop cheap gimmick-ridden marketing of junk, processed food to kids, the government could be too busy thinking that this children's health and NCDs is not a national problem (even when it very much is), the celeb may be too busy making a quick buck out of this — but you? This child is your progeny, your legacy; she must stay healthy and at all costs. Protect them from littering their stomachs — they are, after all, in the growth phase — and the earth. Which food company is paying to pick up their litter, by the way? But you can pick up your child, put her on your lap and say, shh, no discussions or negotiations on this; it's not good for you. Cry all you want but you are too precious for me. Can't let you have poison, sorry.

2. *Coffee Shops in India*

These have become a big hang-out place for kids. Unfortunately, you see them mirroring the same bad habits of the adults — the coffee without sugar or with sweetener and a large pastry to go with it. First of all, help them identify that the coffee shops that rich kids patronise here are for students and people on budgets in their country of origin. About how, let's say, a Starbucks will typically be at a campus, train station, etc., where you either pick stuff to go or use that chair to sit and complete assignments on. That it belongs to a different food environment, and it's not all that posh. But here the cars will get double, even triple parked, the chauffer opens the door and the rich patron walks out, sits, consumes and gets fat. Raising a child in an increasingly global world will mean the responsibility of teaching them different consumption patterns in developing and developed society. Even McDonalds or Burger King, or any fast food chain for that matter, are mostly patronised by the homeless and the poor in those countries, but you will find rich kids eating in them here, even celebrating their birthdays.

And i totally understand that it may not be completely possible to keep them away from chain restaurants, so teach them that this should be a last option, not something aspirational. They should know that what they are consuming is junk, and the least they can do is divide the serving size between four to six people. Not because they are on a budget economically, but in terms of health. Also coffee or chais are both harmful for growing kids; coffee has caffeine and tea has tannins, both interfere with mineral absorption, so expect poor bones, teeth and nails (in addition to bad sleep quality, especially due to caffeine). 'CC, TT,' said one of my ten-year-old clients. And again, i went back to thinking that kids have such smart, quick brains, and even after all these years of working, we haven't come out with this kind of stuff to remind our young clients why not to have coffee or tea.

3) Birthday parties

'Write one section on birthday planning, haan please,' said one of my clients with two children and a third one on the way. She has a boy and a girl, so the third one is not for a boy, so chill. Lots of my clients get very fit and then very pregnant; this is one of those cases. But back to the birthday. 'Don't have it at one of the big pizza and burger chains, that's my standard advice.' 'Arre, please, there are at least fifty birthday parties that a child has to attend per year, minimum, so please write.' 'Really? Fifty?' 'Arre, phir? Dekh, mera social network, uska khud ka, then class, then swimming class, then some family, cousins, bahut social calendar packed hai bachho ka aaj kal.'

So i began to calculate, and mind you i am terrible at calculations. But if there are 365 days in a year, and the kids who have these fifty birthday parties to attend are also the category who have variety for dinner almost every night, holiday for at least two weeks somewhere abroad, accompany their parents to restaurants to eat out a minimum (ekdum minimum) two times a month, then how many days are they really eating home-cooked, local, seasonal, food heritage wala meals? Where does this leave them in terms of NCDs, intolerances, allergies, vitamin D status? The picture is bloody grim. And i am not even calculating the number of times they will just pick up a pastry or a cookie or order in at home.

Anyway, so how must we celebrate birthdays? One of the good ways to celebrate it would be to have a sense of belonging of where we come from. Nothing like food to allow you to dig into where you come from and to let your friends have a taste of it too. So here goes my **good birthday celebration list**:

- A good idea is to have your friends come home, or to a public park or a forest if your city has one (Mumbai has a National Park). And not to a banquet hall, restaurant or the play area of a mall.
- Serve not more than three things — one freshly fried item, one sweet (anything the birthday kid loves) and one wholesome dish. So some combos would be:
  - Samosa – jalebi – poha. Wafers – cakes – veg pulao. Sabudana wada – sheera or halwa – sevaiya upma. Bhajiya – shrikhand – poori aloo bhaji. Kachori – gajjar halwa – biryani. Pav-bhaji – malai sandwich. Suhali – Nolen gur – dal rice. Khandvi – kheer – khichdi.
  - These are just broad ideas; please make your own unique combinations, but keep the menu small.
  - This is the perfect age to teach children that

wealth does not mean having a large spread, but good quality stuff that's local, has the freshest ingredients, is cooked fresh and where no food is wasted. If the kids finish it all and want more, serve dahi-rice or khichdi with papad — they will still rejoice.

- Not to do list: Burgers or chips or anything that has spent months in a cold chain before being fried in oil that is reused like a million times. Or ready to fry at home pattice, French fries and god knows what.
- Limit, and ideally not use, plastic cutlery, bottles, foils, tissues, because we are on the one hand celebrating a birthday, hoping for the long, healthy life of a child, and on the other hand creating immense waste and making the poor child's life difficult on earth.
- Older children can have a perfectly good party even when making bhakris with their hands and creating a mess. Your younger lot can do that too.
- If you are having a party outdoors, like a beach, park, forest, you can bring along banana leaves or plates and bowls made of leaves that you can still buy from any local market in India on pre-order. Make the effort.
- Want more ideas? Have a joint party of four to five kids together, ideally from different backgrounds, different gender and celebrate together. It will help

bring down the fifty parties to fifteen, and will be twice the fun. Sab ka saath, sab ka vikas, kyu?

So, a party that has no pollutants is a good party. That has no wastage, is a good party. Where food is limited but great in quality, is a good party. Where fun not frill is the focus, is a good party. The thing is that we outsource parties because we are getting lazy as parents, and rising incomes allow us to feel that some cartoon character or movie icon theme is a great party. The fact is that no matter how rich or how poor, water, land, forests are shared resources and there needs to be a top-down respect for these resources. If you are the society doyen, the mother of the child who stands first in class, the head of a start-up that struck a billion-dollar deal, the cool CEO, this birthday party is your chance to create an impact. It's your own personal CSR, don't let the opportunity pass.

4) Sports

A child in sports — do they have special needs, especially protein? Well, if your child is a true athlete, then her performance is not coming from what she's eating but from what's eating her from within. An athlete's passion and drive is so unimaginable that you put them in an unreserved railway compartment with rats or cockroaches running over them or fly them business class in an Emirates, and they will do what they will do on the field the next day. No questions asked, no answers needed.

Look at the recently concluded Asian Games: all medals went to the dal-chawal eating sons and daughters of the soil. Now, post medals, they will get endorsements for things from head to toe; that's how it should be as well. It's a valid stream of income for an athlete, but for the consumer to confuse it with the athlete's performance is the problem area. To think that yeh shoes pehen ke, aisa bhaagi. Yeh khake, aisa six mara. Yeh deo se ladki pataya, etc.

A lot of times, parents, especially mothers, worry that their child may not be getting enough nutrients, protein especially, to succeed at their sports. But this worry essentially comes only out of nutritionism. Nutritionism along with nutrition transition leads us to believe that the only way to get enough protein is to eat meat, eggs or gulp down shakes. The more we think like this — this one nutrient ke liye one source, or only a couple of sources — the more we move towards a restricted diet. Oh, i am a vegetarian so now i can only have tofu or paneer and dals for protein. Oh, i am a vegan so only quinoa and soya now. A restricted diet is the opposite of a healthy diet. A healthy diet is a diverse, local (familiar) diet, rich in its nutrient profile and taste; that way it aids in diversity of gut bacteria too.

As for protein sources, you really do get it from everything you are eating. First of all, as discussed earlier, the big stimuli for muscle protein synthesis comes from the gruelling training itself, and the fact that the athlete is always up for the challenge to push harder. Then you have to do a few basic things with food:

i. Stay well hydrated, avoid anything that is dehydrating in nature — chocolate, caffeine, energy drinks, alcohol.
ii. Eat a diverse diet that is in tune with your food heritage, is local and seasonal.
iii. Eat as soon as you are done with training, within twenty minutes of finishing.
iv. Drink water or nimbu sherbet between training if sessions are longer than sixty minutes.
v. Avoid packaged, processed foods and eating late at night.

PROTEIN, INSECTS AND SUSTAINABILITY

The thing is that if your food heritage is a meat- and fish-eating one, keep up with that. And exactly like your grandmom asked you to: a few days on, a few days off. Some fried, some roasted, some curry and always with rice or bhakri, never alone. And in some seasons, totally off, like no fish in monsoon. This is sustainability, sensibility and science rolled into practicality. The rest, as you know, is just food business. Climate change already demands that Europe cut down its meat intake by half by 2050. The human greed for lean protein and omega-3 has destroyed marine bio-diversity already, and the first conference to discuss introducing insects as a source of protein for human consumption has already happened in 2014. Don't confuse this with some Indian tribes eating insects — that's a part of their food heritage. But when you grow insects especially for humans, it is consumption influenced by production (like the almond milk / flour, kale or meat industry currently), and it's invariably unsustainable and sometimes even cruel. Adhering to food heritage ensures that your consumption is based on production (i.e., natural crop cycle), that's future proof and healthy.

With that, what you really need to load up on is sleep. Anyway, children need much more sleep than adults, because this is where all the repair, growth and maintenance work happens. An athletic child needs even more sleep: up to eleven–twelve hours, sometimes even longer. So make room for them to sleep and know that it's perfectly normal that they sleep longer or if they take a short nap post training. If you visit Sports Authority of India (SAI) facilities, you will notice that, when not training, the athletes are all just sleeping or at least lying down on their beds. You may be tempted to call them lazy, but that is really not the case.

It's also important to note that fitness is different from athletics; all athletes are supremely fit, but mostly at that one skill-specific task. In fact, most injuries will come from the fact that they are poor on all-round fitness. They may not be as flexible in the hip, or as mobile as they should be, and there, you snap a hamstring or pull the groin. So yes, get them well-rounded training programs that complement their training in the sport they love, and again, take the pressure off. Keep the focus on having fun and not on winning medals. Medal aaya toh bhi fun, nahi aaya toh bhi. It's still time to figure if this is what they want to do for their living; they are just kids right now. If you push them in a sport to raise your profile within the family, or to get better traction on your social media, it smells of child labour.

So when i get emails from parents saying, my six- or nine- or thirteen-year-old son / daughter is in sports, what should i do, then here's my answer:

i. Allow them to sleep longer.
ii. Allow them to prioritise training over everything else.
iii. Get them to a gym for sport-specific training once a week.
iv. Get them to do yoga asanas, at least the suptapadanghushtasana 1, 2, 3 (Iyengar style)

every time before and after training, and five suryanamaskars every day without fail.

v. Don't post about their achievements on family WhatsApp groups more than once a quarter and on social media more than once a year (this includes your pics in the audience).

A child really is in that divine state where they own nothing and renounce nothing; don't ruin that. Ok, all the faltu bakbak aside — what about diet, because email toh uske liye hi aaya na. So here goes, **meal guidelines for kids in sports**:

i. On rising: one nut + one dry fruit + ghee. For example, date + badam + one teaspoon of ghee (any amount of dates and almonds, no fuss over that). Alternatively, one handful of mixed meva (buy the dry fruits separately and mix them up at home; get the child involved in doing this).
ii. Ragi porridge or anything hot and homemade for breakfast (no bread, no ketchup, no readymade jams, butter) + at least one teaspoon of white butter.
iii. Mid meals — nariyal pani / kokum sherbet / any homemade sherbet.
iv. Pre-training or between training — fresh local fruit or banana or dates or nimbu pani.
v. Post-training, right away — rajgeera chiki (check that it has jaggery and not glucose syrup or stevia or sweetener) or any homemade laddoo. Followed

by the wholesome meal that is next in line based on the time of day, so lunch or dinner or nashta.

vi. Dal-rice or any of the legumes with rice / roti – sabzi for dinner — ensure that the dal or the legumes are pre-soaked before cooking. Also, if using legumes, it's helpful to sprout them in a malmal cloth, by tying it to a tap overnight.

vii. Rub ghee or kokum butter or til oil to the soles of the feet before sleeping (all kids can do this on their own; whether athletes or not, encourage them to do it). It helps with restorative sleep.

viii. If you belong to a meat-, egg-, fish-eating heritage, continue to do so, but as grandma recommended. A few days of the week, not all. Olympic associations across the globe are now reducing the number of weekly meals with meat for their athletes, so your grandma was not just on track but way ahead of her times; don't grudge her for that.

ix. Don't copy the diet of the person who is doing well in that sport, e.g. Virat Kohli or anyone else at all. Your child is unique and on their own growth curve; allow them that. Who knows, they may pretty much have the potential to put these guys behind, so don't come in the way of great and make them good.

x. Lastly, when you feel like switching their diet, ask yourself the important question — is this because of a nutrient — and the answer will just come to you, the confusion will clear and you will know whether to change tracks with the diet or not.

xi. And before i forget, take extra effort to constantly diversify their diet. Change the millet based on the season, only buy fruits and veggies that are local and in season, give them the seasonal halwas and laddoos, even pickles. Don't forget to add the sabzis and fruits that come from the wild and uncultivated category that may last you only a week or fortnight every year. They need to eat it at least four to six times a year.

Know that the portion size of athletic kids is large so don't stress them over it and ask them to eat less. They need the food they are eating and will eat big quantities at one time. Simply remind them to eat slower and ensure that they are not eating any packaged, processed foods.

Points to remember:

i. Some of the veggies that are very useful: raw banana, suran, banana flower, ambadi, nettle, jackfruit.
ii. Fruits: cashew fruit, amla, banana, karvand, ber, jackfruit (cook the seeds of the jackfruit and make a sabzi out of those too), mango, seetaphal, chikoo.
iii. Are there any supplements that are useful? Yes and no. First of all, without the right stimuli of training, love for sport, good sleep, great baseline diet, every

supplement out there will fail. But if you must add some supplements, these are the ones:

- Vitamin B complex with extra B12 — with breakfast or pre training.
- Calcium citrate — bedtime.
- Vitamin C and a multivitamin — post training.
- Iron supplement, preferably in syrup (easy to assimilate) with B complex (once a week).
- Vitamin D, 10–30k IU once every month.
- Gulkand (summer) or chyawanprash (winter) by itself or in milk — once every day or at bedtime.

PROTEIN POWDERS

Bournvita, Complan, Horlicks, Boost, Protinex (sorry if i left any out) — do you need them? Big NO. But do they need sports? Yes. To show themselves as something that can bring sporting greatness. The mother always seated in the stadium, the son performing, she being nervous, then this powder magically putting her at ease and the medal around her son's neck. We have all seen it too often. And yes, if you do read the nutrition label, this is the typical profile you will find: sugars (from really poor sources) being up to three times higher than the amount of protein in those powders.

This is not even counting everything that comes in the GRAS category — the preservatives, emulsifiers, etc. It's nothing short of a daylight heist that these sugar powders have pulled off for years, calling themselves protein-rich, with added vitamins, etc., earning billions from our feelings of inadequacy. So, if you are raising an athlete, let them endorse the product on winning, no judgement; but seeing you serve one of these, will judge, and harshly at that.

Important note: The power of boys and girls in sports

Smriti Mandhana is a prolific cricketer, known for her big sixes, fastest fifties, youngest player to achieve multiple milestones and what have you. She's a pure vegetarian and a powerful hitter but her diet choices hardly make news or influence cricketers or other sports people. Virat Kohli, though, allegedly turned vegan and it made it to the front page of our newspapers. He was apparently a big meat-eater, and i have seen a lot of bonafide pure vegetarians forcing themselves to eat at least eggs, and if not eggs, at least egg whites (coz they can't bear the smell of the yolk) because of that. Now where does his veganism leave them?

The thing that we have to wrap our heads around is

that whether it's Virat Kohli or Smriti Mandhana, these are people too; they are great at what they do, yes, but they are regular folks. They will have certain things in life which influence their diet choices; we should let them be and applaud only when we sit in the stands. And in the meanwhile, know that for every Virat Kohli (who according to unconfirmed news eats this or gives up on that) who dominates the scene, there is a Smriti Mandhana who has stayed loyal to her food heritage and dominates the scene too.

5) NRI kids

To put it plainly, that green card and citizenship has cost you your food system and heritage. It's a trade-off you knew about and it's not all that bad, if you do the basics right. One of my clients headed a PR agency in New York, looked smashing hot but had a very poor body image. She said it stemmed from moving to America when she was in the 6th or 7th standard. Her mother would pack her a dabba of sev-ghatiya or dosa or poha and all the kids would poke fun at her. And the food they ate, she couldn't bring herself to eat — she had moved from a small village in Gujarat straight to NY. So she spent a good part of her school years just not eating. But then that was the 1980s; it's 2018 now and the world has changed.

There's a good chance that your kid learnt of haldi doodh from a café and not from your kitchen, knows about yoga from the university and not home, has chai at Starbucks but doesn't know how to make it at home. The thing is that the West is adopting your grandmom's wisdom and bringing every novel food out there to its kitchens, pantries and even baby milk formulas. We (NRIs), on the other hand, are caught in the middle. If you live in Africa, there's a food heritage to fall back upon — the ugali-githeri-sukumawiki — and you could say that for a fair bit of the Mediterranean region and other Asian countries too. But the US, UK, Australia, have lost their own food heritage, or like one of my American friends says, 'Well, my grandma was eating General Mills' packaged cereals, so when you say eat what grandma ate, do you mean i should eat that?'

NRI kids have the big advantage of using two worlds to their benefit. So here is how you can make right food choices to make the best of both the worlds:

i. The legumes, pulses, grains, millets, spices and the method of cooking should be how it used to be back home, the home you grew up in.
ii. And let the fruits, vegetables, dairy and meat be from the local farmers' market.
iii. Get them to eat one home-cooked Indian meal a day, don't expect them to love it. It's not because they don't love Indian but because all kids of all nationalities don't like (or like very rarely) what is cooked at home. They must eat it, nevertheless, to ensure that the palate doesn't change to accepting

only ultra-processed food as good food and to keep the gut bacteria thriving.

SENDING KIDS ABROAD

'i am sending him to London now,' said one of my clients to me about her twenty-one-year-old son. She wanted him to get a little independent, she explained. This is a common trend and you must have seen it all around you. Sixteen- to twenty-year-olds going abroad for studies; mothers and fathers flying out with them, helping them find an apartment, settling them down, getting their kitchens up and running, giving them a bottomless pit of a credit card, etc. Then staying back for fifteen–twenty days with them and doing FaceTime with them for twenty minutes twice a day after coming back. 'How is this supposed to get him independent, darling,' i asked my client. 'Ruj,' she offered, 'Sunday ko chauffeur nahi aata hai udhar, so he will have to walk and be on his own.' 'Really, your twenty-one-year-old little thing, walking all by himself in central London, hard work!' Ok, i didn't say that aloud. But the question is, must we raise them to be entirely incapable of being independent while they are still here in school and at home? You send them abroad, wherever they go, it's a compromise on the food system, their gut bacteria and long-term health. Keep them home at least till they graduate and get them to eat good, home-cooked meals right here. Send them on the four holidays i listed earlier to make them independent, teach them a sport — there's a lot to do right here to build independence. Again free gyan from my experience of meeting all kinds of people, but the happiest and the healthiest kids are the ones who are self-reliant, and wealth cannot guarantee that. In fact, most times it takes away from that. And like one of my ex-advertising clients said to me, cash is a poor substitute for upbringing. There you go. Independent in your chatra chaya please. Then they are free to go anywhere they want. From self-reliance comes shanti, and from there comes sukh for all involved. Don't forget that we are the original *sarve bhavantu sukhinaha* culture.

6) Fussy eater

You are raising them in 2018–19 — it will be a surprise if they are *not* fussy eaters. They are living in a world of endless options and around people who refer to food by its nutrients and not by its name. It's disrespectful, btw, to not call people by their name and the same with food. *Annam na nindayat* is one of the preliminary vows of a good, honourable life. Never criticise food. To teach that, practice that. Not entirely related to this, but one of my friends who grew up in a village in Punjab told me that they would call Bihari workers 'chawl'. 'What's that?' 'Arre, chawl, like kadhi-chawl, that's rice.' It was a way of looking down upon the poor rice-eating farm workers by the wheat-eating farm owners. So no name for them, just chawl. And hum log, these days, don't even call it rice, but carbs or starch. Human stupidity is truly infinite.

Alright, so how do you deal with a fussy eater? Very simply, by adopting the basic rules and upholding some basic good behaviour yourself. Like not taking the phone to the loo. In health studies, there is something called as clustering of lifestyle behaviours and, in my observation, parents who take phones to the loo or (walking on eggshells here) update their status more than once a day, have kids who are fussy eaters.

And that's because you are missing out on observing something very basic. That the kid is only fussy about homemade food but always has an appetite for ultra-processed food. Just this morning at the farm, one of our kids from the 'Sonave community farming project' told his dad that he didn't want to eat the rice that we had served at 11 a.m. 'Come on, beta, eat now,' said the dad. 'See, how nicely all your friends are eating and do you know it's already 11 o'clock, time to eat.' When the kid didn't relent, the dad announced, 'Ok, i am not going to stop anywhere on the road.' 'No, no we have to go to Decathlon on the way,' says the kid. The dad nods, they need to buy something. But right next to their stop is a McDonalds, and how exactly do you think this is going to end? So i intervened and said, 'You know, carry the rice and whenever the kid is hungry offer it to him.' 'Yeh achha idea hai,' the dad said teasingly to the kid. Because he had realised what the kid was up to, and even if we say things like, i won't stop anywhere on the way, close to McDonalds the kid gets hungry, please please this one time papa, he will say. Heart will melt, happy meal will be consumed, but no one's going to be happy or at least healthy in the long term.

The thing is that, once again, the junk food industry guns for our kids and they are too young to resist, but we must use age-old techniques to protect them. Manipulating parents into giving in is easy for kids, but you must learn to hold your own. This is what Appa would do:

i. First of all, give no option to say no when lunch or dinner is served.
ii. And if the kid really says that they cannot, for whatever reason, bring themselves to eat right now, then whenever later, an hour later, four hours later, they get hungry, offer them the exact same food.

Basically, don't give them any wriggle room. If i was hungry for wafers later and had skipped lunch, Appa would sing, '*Bhakri taji ho athva shili, deyi deyi bhuke chya weli.*' It's an abhanga or a devotional song to Vitthal. The devotee says that i don't want much in life, just a basic meal of either a fresh or stale bhakri (millet roti, quite the rage these days but a standard meal for farmers since time immemorial), but only when i am hungry. With a song on his lips, he conveyed everything that i needed to hear:

a) *i know what you are trying to do here.*
b) *Bhakri (or anything that was made for lunch, a basic meal) is all you will get.*
c) *Enjoy the simple joys of life to lead a good life.*
d) *The most basic of meals is also a divine blessing — don't treat it with disrespect.*
e) *Learn to eat when food is served, with everybody.*
f) *You are not the first kid i have raised — don't try this with me again.*

Sometimes, all we lack is self-belief. Once you are confident that you are putting your foot down for the child's long-term health, you will feel more empowered to sing this song. And you will have a version of this by every saint and in every language. Also, don't worry if you are a poor singer — the kid will eat on time simply to prevent being tortured by your singing.

Part 2c — Health Issues/ NCDs

1) Fat kid / Thin kid

Putting these two together because that's how we need to view them. First of all, your kid's size or weight is no one's business, not even yours. If the kid is running around all day, enthusiastic about school, eats independent of gadgets, sleeps on time, you have nothing to worry about, regardless of size and weight. The diverse races and ethnicities that we belong to makes it impossible for the poor kid to comply or fall into the percentile that you desperately want him / her to belong to. But a healthy child or an unhealthy one can be easily spotted by parents, even neighbours.

So track real stuff that defines health: the kid is largely happy and sometimes fussy; screams, runs and laughs at the same time; generally makes for an enthu cutlet and has a deep interest in one or two things? You are safe; don't worry about weight or size. And if you see an unhappy, apprehensive, low energy kid, then worry. Your first line of treatment should always be introspection, and then after that do the basics — food, exercise, sleep, saying no to junk, binge watching, endless lying around — and do not fear about reaching out to a professional for help. But don't put them on a weight loss diet or give them tonics to increase weight.

All that kids who are at both extremes need is higher bone density, more muscle mass and less adipose tissue. And that is easily achievable with all the rules listed out in the book. So at both extremes, you will need play, wholesome meals, sleep hygiene and really just that. And a little bit of backing off, like not pinching their thighs and saying, 'pudgy like mumma's', or tapping stomachs to say 'round like daddy', or 'sukdi like dadi'.

Important note — Metabolic health

What really counts is the metabolic health of the child. That is why scientists even came up with terms like 'FOTI' (Fat outside, Thin inside) and 'TOFI' (Thin outside, Fat inside) to describe the importance of metabolic health over weight. Here is a quick list of metabolic health parameters that matter:

i) Good sleep quality: Falls asleep almost at the same time every night and has an undisturbed sleep through the night. Doesn't find the need to sleep endlessly over weekends / holidays (an hour extra is fine).
ii) High energy levels through the day: Looks forward to playing outdoors as soon as he / she is back from school

or after finishing homework. Doesn't feel lethargic or need tea / coffee to feel enthusiastic.

iii) Good digestion / excretion: Generally, keeps a fixed potty time and doesn't take too long doing it. Doesn't have frequent issues of bloating, acidity or constipation / loosies.

iv) Good immunity levels: Doesn't fall sick often, especially with each change of season or just because someone in the class has cold and cough. Is able to easily adjust to new places when on a holiday.

v) No PMS or period pain: Effortless period, without any physical trouble or awkwardness. Doesn't feel angry, irritable, sick during periods.

Also, if they are around puberty or around eight to twelve, whether it's a girl or a boy, expect a bit of change, and even a little roundish appearance around the stomach. That's just all the DHEA (a hormone) turning into estrogen in our girls and testosterone in our boys. They are simply transitioning, don't make a big deal out of it; change in body composition during this phase is natural. And that's why all the more reason you should keep your eye on the basics; that's the foundation they need to flourish and fly.

And if others around you want to judge you for the size of your kid or the lack of it, let them; it's a free world and everyone is entitled to their share of time pass. Don't alter the kid's food or body composition to appease anyone else. Health comes in all sizes. And the thing i worry about often these days is that if all our kids are fed the same food, read the same book, speak in the same language (angrezi, angrezi), then what are we raising but prototypes of each other. Whether it's language, food or sizes, humanity lies in diversity not uniformity.

2) Poor immunity

The rich kids seem to have the poorest immunity. They fall sick with every change in season, for every reason and occasion. And these are the exact same kids where there's fussing over hygiene, sanitisers, etc.

One of my clients showed me a pic and said, 'See this.' It was a pic of a little foot. i looked at it and drew a blank. 'Can't you see?' she asked. i squinted my eyes, twisted my neck and zoomed into the picture to get a closer look. 'What am i looking at?' i asked myself. 'Is this some gift that someone made in gold that looks like a real human foot? Did her boy just celebrate a birthday or something?' Annoyed with the time i was taking, she snatched the phone out of my hand, zoomed into the picture and showed me exactly one grey spot on the ball of the big toe. 'Look at that filthy, dusty, bedroom of ours. My babu walks and gets all dirty; this is every day. i have horrible staff at home,' she exclaimed. She had sent the same pic to the paediatrician and she was rather miffed that he said this was not the reason for her boy's frequent allergies or weak immunity; that, in fact, this didn't qualify as dirty. 'All i want to do is raise my son in a good home, but the maids are always plotting against me,' she said. 'They are my MIL's old-timers.' 'The MIL may hate you but won't bring harm on her grandchild, grandson that too,' i tried to reason but to no avail.

At the Delhi airport once, while standing in a long-winding queue for the boarding gate, i saw a little kid crawl out. Bare hands, toes curled up, curious, this little six- to eight-month-old was free to roam the world, and brought a smile to everyone's faces at the Indira Gandhi havai adda. His mother stood in the queue, wearing a saree, head covered, looking not even a wee bit worried about her kid's adventure. 'Naam kamayega bada hoke, raised by a strong, fearless woman,' i said to my partner. 'Joint family ma'am?' i asked the lady. 'Yes,' she nodded. Nosy that i am, 'Twenty-eight people?' i prodded. 'Fifty-six,' she replied.

So why am i telling you this? Because the mother's stress often gets to a child — something that every paediatrician will agree with. And it's important to not sweat the small stuff, literally. A little bit of dust and dirt will do no damage to a kid; they are a part of growing up, in fact. Here's a list of other things that should be in place for a strong immunity:

i. A homemade achaar, morambas or khata-meetha chutneys for the kids. Have one teaspoon a day with roti or bhakri or paratha or a wholesome meal, to keep the gut resilient and maintain gut integrity.

ii. A mixture of jaggery, ghee, a little dry ginger and a pinch of haldi post lunch and dinner. Small, nail-size laddoos, like a mouth-freshner, not a big ball.

iii. Well-cooked sabzis, well-soaked dals, well-sprouted legumes when cooking.

iv. Regular filtered water for cooking, cleaning, drinking, bathing, shampooing. No bathing kids in mineral water or whatever.

v. Limit use of refrigerator and feed fresh meals.

vi. A multivitamin syrup with breakfast or lunch.

vii. No anger, stress, smoking, alcohol around the kid.

viii. Don't unnecessarily medicate or use antibiotics. Remind yourself of the basics, like a cold takes seven days to recover, a viral cannot be treated with antibiotics, and falling sick a couple of days or up to ten days in one year is totally ok. Normal life.

ix. Bedtime and wake-up time fixed and strictly adhered to. And the basics again, you should be up before the kid, or at least a responsible member of the family should be.

x. Strong familial relationships where you can depend on each other. And when there are problems and misunderstandings — because there always will be — an open and honest chat with the adult involved. But at all points of time, no sly remarks, no playing politics and scoring points over the kid's food, health and well-being.

3) Fatty liver

One of the fast-spreading NCDs amongst children. At one time a fatty liver (inflamed liver with abnormally high storage of triglycerides; a type of fat) was limited to only adults who were regular consumers of alcohol. Now, though, you can see it in kids as young as six years old. Their sedentary lifestyles, high consumption of packaged food and irregular bedtimes is to be blamed here. i have seen parents of kids with non-alcoholic fatty liver disease, or NASH as it's called, really at a loss as to how exactly to help the child and then playing that blame game: 'Kuch bhi bana do, isko two-minute Maggi noodles hi chahiye', 'Kyu piya aapne kal cold drink, mamma ne mana kiya tha na? You never listen to me'.

Chalo, chhodo yeh sab and you listen to me. First of all, wake up and smell the coffee. We are raising our children in an obesogenic environment, and that is the major contributor to the NCDs in kids, and you as an individual are not the only one responsible. Government, policymakers, industries, advertising, and so many more play an active role in your child's health. You know this by now, but here is a quick recap of the obesogenic environment and what we can do about it:

i. Poor planning of towns and cities, no open spaces, parks or greenery. Don't chabao the brain of the kid, get together as a society, talk to the local MLA and ask them to help make walking and not driving the default option. If you are a politician and reading this, come on sir / ma'am, our kids, your future voters, deserve better.

ii. No regulation on marketing junk food to children. If you are involved in ad making or belong to the IAS, sirs and ma'ams, our time starts now. Childhood obesity is a ticking bomb and needs policymakers to intervene and diffuse that threat.

iii. And then there's pollution, effluents reaching our water resources without adequate treatment, landfills that suffocate every living being within a five-km radius. So if you are a business baron or industrialist, your time to act is now. Clean air is a human right, and when you deny your future consumers that, profits will dip, karma will catch up. Ok, maybe you don't believe in karma, but reduced human capital due to sickness means that people are not really interested in buying your products or you will lose productivity due to employee sickness and lose money to insurance.

Ok, i don't know if i convinced the politician, policymaker or the industrialist, but i do hope that i have convinced the parent within that this isn't a carb, protein, fat, calories issue. It is NOT just a lifestyle problem, even though it gets categorised like that medically. It is a social, economic, political, policy, ecological problem. And it will need a multi-pronged approach. In the meanwhile, there's a lot you can do, starting from — you can stop blaming the kid, you can stop thinking that you are a failure as a parent. Now in terms of lifestyle, here's the list:

i. Sleep, the most crucial of all factors to ensure that all organs, especially liver, kidney, heart and brain work at their optimum. A fatty liver means that the liver is holding on to too many triglycerides. Leave this unaddressed for too long and it can land you with a blood sugar problem too. So what the doctor told you is correct, except that they forgot to add that what works like medicine for this problem is sleep, not drugs. And the very basic of sleep hygiene — so basic that you may miss the magic — is sleeping and waking up at fixed times every day. If you just do this over and over, three months at a stretch, you will see the wonders it works on the kid's health. Once a week, you can let them change the timing by an hour, but no more. Sleep is medicine, by-heart that. It's gonna fight the underlying insulin resistance and the circulating triglycerides; no messing with this.

ii. Five suryanamaskars a day, every day, holiday and Sunday included, ideally before school or at sunrise or sunset.

iii. Ninety minutes of play and activity. This is crucial and there are no alternatives. You can do a mix of structured and unstructured play; it's important that the kid loves this. All ninety minutes at one go ideally, and post school. School sports period and recess doesn't count. Dance class, sports coaching, just playing downstairs, gym, swimming, cycling — a mix of these or one of these or all of these. Ensure that this gets done.

iv. Limit gadgets and screens of all kinds to thirty minutes max per day. And no extension on weekends. You can exclude the school work or an odd movie that you watch from the thirty minutes, but other than that strictly monitor. And let me state the obvious — no screen during meals and no screen in the bedroom.

v. Nothing out of a packet. No ketchup, dips, crackers, biscuits, nachos, tortillas, nothing, zilch. No colas, no coffees, no chocolates, no chais. No ordering out, pizzas or whatever, and no, it doesn't help that you ordered the low-cal, low-fat version. And also, no ready-made attas — buy your own gehu and mill it at a local chakki. Basically, it's not about consumption of fat or sugar but where it comes from. And the more processed form it comes in, the further away its origins are from your kitchens and your farms. What is not grown in the farm and not cooked in the kitchen is a recipe for disease, irrespective of what the label reads. So stay as far away from it as possible. Ultra-processed food in any and all quantities is a problem for both circulating fats and blood sugar.

vi. Eat millet, makhan and chutney — one meal of this combo, every day, either for breakfast, lunch, dinner or between 4 and 6 p.m. One of the main meals needs to be something that grounds the kid in their food heritage, re-orients their palate preferences from the processed stuff and helps them improve insulin sensitivity and keeps the circulating triglycerides low. The essential fat in the makhan, or ghee if you prefer, the micronutrients in the chutney, the nutrient profile in the millet will do just that.

Know that fatty liver (or the elevated blood sugars — pre-diabetes or diabetes — that may show up with it) is very much a reversible condition. Yes, it's preventable too, but in case you have landed up here, you can easily retrace the steps back to health if you as parents and as a family take the lead. The kid's job is then just to follow your example. And do engage with a doctor who is aware that it is a reversible condition and one that doesn't freak you out but backs your efforts to correct your lifestyle.

4) Diabetes

Everything that goes for a fatty liver pretty much goes for diabetes too. And the note above and what we will discuss now is applicable for both Type 1 and Type 2 of diabetes. First of all, i work with a whole lot of kids now who are

Type 2 diabetic. It starts with the same kind of thing: high circulating levels of insulin (hyperinsulinemia, as it's called) and triglycerides. Along with this there are elevated blood sugars and low levels of vitamin B12, vitamin D and haemoglobin. This invariably seems to happen somewhere around their puberty (the period seems to trigger it in the girls), somewhere between eleven to fourteen years. For me, the heartbreak is often meeting the parents; the kids are just fine, optimism comes naturally to them. Within minutes, they are giggling, they make up their minds to tackle this menace one day at a time. The parents, on the other hand, seem even more fearful about the fact that the kid is not stressing about the condition now. They tend to feel that darenge nahi toh karenge kaise! Karenge, samajh gaye iss liye karenge. Fear has no role to play, nor is it a motivator.

Anyway, it's not very clear what seems to trigger it. Is it the flux of hormones during puberty or is it the fact that they are babies born to mommies who received treatment for their pregnancy. The pumped hormonal status of the mother during conception and through the pregnancy has a role to play here too, says my gut. Because all this is bound to change the microbiota diversity for the kid, and then, of course, the fact that most of these births are not vaginal, further limits the bacterial eco-system. The packaged, processed food, and the inactive, gadget-friendly kid, is not the complete picture; there's a lot in the background that we are missing here.

But the thing is, if there's diabetes, get a doctor who says, i will take you off the drug (Type 2) or regulate the dose (Type 1), as the numbers get better; not the one who says, it's lifelong now, and the aim of allopathy is to make life easy. Uh, for who exactly? It's not easy for the kid who's taking the meds and getting driven on the guilt trip for wanting even aloo sabzi. Anyway, i am happy to report that there are doctors who do support kids, and we had one kid with a HbA1c of 11.6 go off drugs (all drugs) within four months of eating right and with the doctor cheering all along. The young breed of doctors are enthu, so are the ones who are seventy+, who have more than witnessed the routine of people starting on 500mcg of a hypoglycaemic drug, going on 2000mcg in a matter of two to three years. So find a good person instead of the best doctor. Get what i am saying?

Toh bachha kya kare? Everything listed in the list above for fatty liver, and these too:

i. Homemade dahi or chaas — either by itself or with a meal or as a dish like khandvi, kadhi, ukad, etc.
ii. Handful of cashews or aliv laddoo — once a day, essentially include an iron-rich source in the baseline diet.
iii. Ghee in every meal — at least four to six teaspoons every day, without fear, without guilt.
iv. Vitamin B12, vitamin D and calcium citrate supplements.

v. Once a week strength training (you can refer to *Don't Lose Out, Work Out*). Ask the trainer to monitor for correct technique and ensure that the kid doesn't reach failure (a point where they cannot do the next repetition).

vi. Stay well hydrated. Encourage the kid to drink water in between play and to eat a banana as soon as they are done playing.

Important note

Once their blood sugar is stable, don't worry about the condition striking back. A boy i worked with for around three years, from his 8th to 11th standard (he is twenty-six years old now), recently messaged me that his insulin, which used to be 24 when we started, is now 8. The beauty of sustainable diets and lifestyle modification is that it keeps you healthy in the long term. And it does that because eating right and making exercise a way of life feels good.

5) Oral health

Often undervalued, but one that has long-term health implications for the kid. Dr Sandesh Mayekar, the man behind the most beautiful smiles in the film industry, is in that lovely stage of his life where he has more than enough laurels to rest on, but still has a packed day at work to both earn and to lend himself to the good of the society. 'First decade, no decay', is one of his pet projects, and obviously the drive behind this are the little kids on his chair with root canals, chronic cavities, bleeding gums.

The thing is, we think that various organs of our body are ranked in a hierarchy like 12th standard marks. So the one with max marks goes to medicine, uske niche engineering, uske niche commerce, etc., but that's not quite how human physiology works. Oral health, especially, is as much a sign of systemic dysfunction or critical to health as the heart is. So if the milk teeth are getting a cavity, the gums are bleeding or the real tooth is just cracking, your mouth is screaming for you to clean up your act.

A study on aboriginals in Australia showed how they had good teeth and great health until the white man came in with the gun and packaged food. Their original diet was pretty much like our food heritage — diverse, local and seasonal; millets, pulses, occasional meat, fruits and veggies. That changed to the aspirational breakfast cereal, muffin, processed meat — the Western diet as it is called — and the accompanying low activity, classic nutrition transition. Today, the aboriginals, once the owners of the land and a healthy, thriving populace, are reduced to a marginalised community that suffers from metabolic diseases.

A bit like how anything desi was mocked: 'Badan ke liye doodh badam aur daton ke liye koyla?' The same company will today sell you the same toothpaste with activated charcoal; you will have cereal for breakfast, chocolate for celebration and cavities for teeth. Get the picture? Go back to eating minimally processed food — stuff that comes from the farms and gets cooked in your kitchens, that's how you maintain oral health.

The colas, chocolates, cereals are the obvious stuff to avoid, but there's more to this story. One of my clients told me that their two-year-old's teeth were very poor though they only fed him healthy stuff. 'Like what?' i asked. 'Only meat and veggies, only brown rice, only cakes made from almond flour, etc. Sugar toh he has not even touched,' they said, 'but yet the teeth and the gums are in poor condition.' The doctor had asked them to change his diet but they were like 'what can be healthier than this?'

Well, the healthiest thing you can do is not think in terms of sugar, carb, protein, fat, but local, seasonal and food heritage. The thing is, as you cut out the sugar, and even wholesome food, in the name of cutting carbs, you have done so at the cost of increasing the phytic acid intake of the kid. That brown rice, those oats, the almond flour and the monotony of this day in and day out, demineralises the poor kid's teeth and damages the oral health. So we just have to apply our common sense and know that cakes are bad. They don't get any better because they are made with almond flour and without sugar. They can be made of anything, but it must be something that the kid eats rarely. Nothing makes junk healthy. No jumla please.

So here's what the kid must eat and do to ensure that oral

health, which is similar to overall health, is well maintained:

i. A local, seasonal, fresh fruit every day — not the kiwi, blueberry, star fruit variety.

ii. White butter every day — to help restore the mineral density in the teeth.

iii. Millets or rice with legumes every day.

iv. Stay adequately hydrated and end meals with chaas or buttermilk.

v. Eat meals slowly, mouth rinsed post meals.

vi. Rethink the use of special kid toothpastes, as they are loaded with sugar.

Essentially, the question that parents must ask themselves when choosing food for kids is — how come i am seeing this on the shelf of the supermarket? Is this about consumption driven by production? Like in the mango season, you will see more mangoes and people eating those. Or is it production driven by consumption? Like a lot of almond milk and cakes with almond flour (flourless as they are often called), or broccoli or quinoa, where clearly consumption is driven by production. So wherever it's the latter, use discretion, because you can't flood markets with large amounts overnight without using unhealthy production practices which will then influence gut bacteria and those in the mouth too. To cut a long story short, eat stuff where its consumption is driven by production. Banana over kiwi. Rice over quinoa. Occasional cake instead of a nut bar or almond cake.

Part 2d — Frequent Illnesses: Quick Pointers

1) Constipation

i. Dahi bhaat or khichdi for both lunch and dinner with at least two teaspoons of ghee.
ii. Ragi kheer or dosa.
iii. Water, nariyal pani and nimbu sherbet with kalanamak through the day.
iv. No straining on the pot, and preferably use an Indian toilet.
v. End lunch / dinner with a local banana.
vi. Ask the kid to externally apply coconut oil or homemade makhan to the anus area.
vii. Supplement with vitamin B12 and especially with vitamin D if constipation is frequent.
viii. Encourage daily play and adherence to bedtime routine.
ix. Rub soles with ghee, kokum butter or til oil before sleeping.

2) Loose motions

i. Do not force-feed the child; allow them to go hungry if they don't feel like eating.
ii. Encourage them to stay well hydrated and sip on water throughout the day.
iii. Nariyal pani or any local sherbet with kalanamak, two to three times a day.
iv. Ghee-roasted makhana (at home) with kalanamak and jeera or black pepper, as per taste.
v. Ask them to eat a banana.
vi. Rice konjee, pej or khichdi or dahi rice for both lunch and dinner.
vii. Avoid sun exposure to prevent dehydration.
viii. Avoid meat, eggs and milk while they are still recovering.

3) Cold and cough

i. Gargle with hot water with salt every morning and night.
ii. Give a teaspoon of local or forest honey post meals (buy locally when on trips — government-run shops and farmers' markets are two good places to source honey).
iii. Haldi doodh works wonders. Add just a pinch of nutmeg, sugar or jaggery to taste.
iv. Small nail-size balls of ghee, jaggery, haldi, dry

ginger (in equal amounts) two to three times a day; anytime is ok.

v. Make khichdi with a bit of dry ginger and jeera and give it to them for dinner.

4) Flu

i. Sip on water through the day — that's very important.
ii. B complex and vitamin C with breakfast or lunch.
iii. Sheera or suji halwa for breakfast or lunch.
iv. Make a nice besan or nariyal rava laddoo for the kid to eat.
v. Ask them what they feel like eating, make that at home. Indulge them a bit.

5) Travel sickness and nausea

i. First of all, tell them that this is nothing to be embarrassed about.
ii. Encourage them to be well hydrated for the journey (tell them it's cool to pee on the road if needed. Also stop at petrol pumps which have decent loos. If you have girls, ensure that they don't learn our unhealthy habit of not drinking water because we are too shy about the need to pee).
iii. Take a tiny drop of coconut oil on your little finger and rub it clockwise in their ears and nostrils, fifteen to twenty minutes before the journey or while leaving from home.

iv. Jam-bread, bread-butter, chivda, sev mamra, are good options to eat while travelling. Light and not very high, or devoid of fibre.
v. Stay away from packaged and processed foods, but they can have three to five sips of cola if they feel like throwing up during the journey.
vi. Sit facing the direction of travel, wear very loose and comfortable clothes. Cover chest, neck and ears, if very cold. Avoid sitting in direct sunlight. So carry a light shawl with which they can cover themselves from both too much sun or wind.
vii. Carry khaddi shakkar and ask them to suck on it during take-off / landing.

6) UTI

Not quite uncommon with kids these days and can be quite painful when it happens.

i. Clean, fresh, cotton underwear with elastic that doesn't hurt.
ii. Loose clothes that allow the vagina, testicles to breathe.
iii. Kokum sherbet, bel sherbet, nimbu sherbet, any local sherbet (add sabja seeds to the sherbet) that keeps them hydrated and has the micronutrients that their body needs to heal.
iv. Enough water through the day so that urine is clear in colour.

v. Preferably use the Indian toilet at all times, but definitely when you are using public loos.
vi. No using tissues or dabbing all the time after defecating or urinating. Use water for the big job and you really need nothing post doing sussu.
vii. Include home-set curd and buttermilk at least once a day.
viii. Include a B-complex syrup with breakfast.
ix. End meals (lunch and dinner) with a teaspoon of gulkand.
x. Include coconut water and coconut in your diet.

7) Period pain

i. First things first, it's not normal. Periods should not be painful at all — at worst, a mild inconvenience because of frequent changing of pad / tampon.
ii. It's biology at work, nothing to be embarrassed or shy about. If you stain a bedsheet, panty, seat / sofa cover, it's cool. Feel bad for the people who may make fun of you for it, or judge you for that.
iii. Keep up with playing regularly even during your period: ninety minutes per day is critical.
iv. Start your day with soaked black raisins and one to three strands of kesar a week before your period, during your period and keep it up for a week after also.

v. Eat aliv laddoo, one every day, one week prior to your periods. You can eat the entire month too, no problem, and you can do this irrespective of age.

vi. Mix jaggery with two to three dhania seeds and ghee and have it immediately after lunch and dinner.

vii. Avoid junk food and excess tea, coffee, chocolate on all days, but especially during periods.

viii. Expect appetite to fluctuate; you may either feel like eating much more or less than usual, or feel hungry at unusual times; it's ok. Feed your body as per the call of the stomach.

ix. Drink a nice cooling sherbet every day, but surely on period days.

x. Eat rajgeera chiki, homemade laddoo or halwa for at least the first three days of your period.

xi. Make tubers like suran, arbi, sweet potato, etc. a part of your weekly diet and surely eat one of them during your periods. Ask them to be made the way you like them.

xii. If your breasts hurt or inner thighs feel reddish or burn, or very simply you feel annoyed or irritated, you could be running low on vitamins B6, B1 and B12. A vitamin B supplement daily will help greatly.

xiii. Include legume preparations like usal and sundals in your weekly diet.

xiv. If period pain persists, lie in suptabaddhakonasana with a bolster to support your back, this will greatly ease the flow and the cramps.

xv. Take a calcium supplement — calcium citrate preferably (easy on the stomach) — daily or every other day at bedtime.

xvi. Take an extra calcium tablet on the day of the period if there is pain (my guess is there won't be, if you keep up with everything as discussed above).

xvii. Don't forget to keep up with your regular play and sports throughout the month.

xviii. Stay well hydrated at all times.

xix. Adhere to a bedtime routine.

xx. In terms of routine life, know that there is nothing that you can or cannot do, just because you have your periods.

Epilogue: A Manifesto for a Healthy Future

The three stakeholders — parents, schools and policymakers — working together to ensure a healthy environment for children. That's a future we should aspire for.

Parents

1. Ensure that all members of the family work in the kitchen and do small tasks at home themselves.
2. As a family, practice 'internet fasting' atleast once a month. Also, no TV dinners and other gadgets during meals and an hour before sleeping.
3. Take children to a local farm atleast twice a year. Ensure that they can identify local fruit trees, seasonal vegetables and know the harvest time of at least rice, tur dal and sugarcane.
4. Raise the child to be able to speak fluently in their mother tongue and at least one other local language. Especially during meal times. The UN has declared 2019 as the international year of indigenous languages.
5. Holiday and party responsibly.

SCHOOLS

1. Have a small plot of land to farm on, even a small patch with veggies will do. Include farming / agriculture in the syllabus.
2. Encourage children to bring and distribute family heritage recipes on birthdays. Make food policies that encourage traditional / local food. Include these in your school menu.
3. Invest wisely in PT teachers and have a compulsory sports or free play class every day.
4. Work with local politicians to get safe cycling / walking lanes for atleast a kilometre around the school. Discourage parents from dropping their kids in private vehicles right in front of the school gate.
5. Have an annual grandparents day to facilitate an open and freewheeling discussion on food, culture, life in general.

POLITICIANS AND POLICYMAKERS

1. Bring in legislation that stops junk food companies from targeting their advertisements to children, using children in their ads, regulates the timing of the ads and use of toys and other offers in their ads. Limit junk food ads in the same manner as tobacco and alcohol ads are (without the loopholes). No junk food ads on public transport.

2. Reserve open spaces for girls on specific day(s) of the week.
3. Implement 'junk food tax' and hold the food industry accountable for collecting and recycling their plastic packaging. Work towards making the 'healthy choice the easy choice'.
4. Plant local trees to beautify new / revamped roads and big projects like airports, etc.
5. Rethink subsidies for chemical fertilisers and instead support native methods of agriculture and local produce, especially the NUS (neglected and underutilised species) and NTFP (non-timber forest produce) categories.

Appendix

What, When and How to Eat

Group 1: Foods you should eat daily / weekly

These are foods that you can have daily (or once a week) as part of your diet. There are about thirty in the list, and for each food there are at least five different ways to prepare it in your kitchen / region, giving a total of minimum 150 food options. Next time your parents say they don't know what healthy and tasty stuff to make, show them this list.

Food	How to eat	Special notes
Rice and wheat	• Can be a part of the main meal and repeated more than once in the day. • You can make rotis out of both rice and wheat. • Rice can also be turned into a kanji (soup), or even mixed with milk or dahi and had as a meal.	• Choose hand-pounded or single polished rice over brown rice. • Choose the local variety, one that grows abut 100–160 km around you.

Food	How to eat	Special notes
	• Atta laddoos or poli or roti laddoos are a good idea too. • Most Indian breakfasts — idli, dosa, upma, sattu, poha, ghavan, paratha — are versions of rice and wheat.	• Buy from farms or small cooperatives, avoid pre-packed rice. E.g.: the large gunny bags are better than the industrialised packaged rice. • And the rice or wheat that comes from only one field, called single origin, is the best.*
Millets	• Have either as a bhakri or roti. There's a special way to make this millet bhakri, where the dough is kneaded in hot water and then the roti is pressed on the hands, instead of rolled with a pin. • You can have as chiki or laddoo as well — rajgeera chiki is especially healthy. • Like a porridge for breakfast or even cooked like a kheer, halwa. • Thalipeeth is also a popular way to integrate millets in the daily diet.	• Use them as per season: – Jowar in summer and year-round. – Bajra in winter. – Kuttu in winter. – Makai in winter. – Ragi in summer, monsoon and year-round. – Jhangora or samo chawal or varai kheers on special occasions. • Important: These days you get packaged pancakes, cakes, cereals, etc., made of millets. These are methods of selling 'nutrients' in the millets for a profit.

* This and the two points above are common for all the foods in the table.

Food	How to eat	Special notes
		It's like the current turmeric craze. When you use an ancient grain or millet but do not follow its food heritage or cooking practices, you don't quite get the nutritional and health benefits.
Pulses and legumes	• Main meal as curry, sabzi, usals, sundal, chilla, dosa, idli, sambar, dal. • As a mid meal: Besan laddoo, sattu, moong dal halwa, sundal. • Mid meal, as raw peanuts / boiled whole peanuts or til chiki or laddoo, both as garnishing in a main meal. • Often turned into dry chutneys as well. • Used to be stored as an insurance against drought and famine in the old times.	• India had more than 65,000 varieties of pulses and we have lost out on most of them. • Pulse is a dry legume. • Global nutrition bodies now regard these as both protein and vegetables because they make for a good source of amino acids, vitamins, minerals and fibre. • So don't force kids to have veggies if they are having these. • Include at least twelve different varieties of pulses in your diet. • Buy loose from a local vendor, not a branded packet.

Food	How to eat	Special notes
		• Avoid using soda while preparing. Soak overnight. And have with traditional recipes and accompaniments for optimum assimilation.
Fresh fruits	• Can be eaten first thing before going to school, post school, post playing, in between games (like banana). • Mango, banana and jackfruit can be had with main meals or even as a late-night meal if studying at night. • Mid meal — whole fruit, fresh fruit milkshake.	• Buy fresh, seasonal and local. • Avoid fruit that is non-native and comes from another country / continent, like kiwi, etc. • Eating a fruit is always preferable to juicing it. As long as you have teeth, chew the fruit.
Fresh, cooked vegetables	• Eat a diversity of sabzis, like turai, pumpkin, dudhi, suran, etc. — all the forgotten, but very local, native and rich-in-nutrient varieties. Eaten as part of the main meal.	• Avoid vegetables that are non-native and come from another country / continent, like broccoli, different coloured bell peppers, asparagus, etc. Applicable even if they are now grown in India. (Because this happens at the cost of local, lesser known vegetables and fruits, and use tons of chemical fertilisers).

Food	How to eat	Special notes
	• Suran, sweet potato, etc., even eaten as mid meal. Can make for a good pre-game meal. • Ensure that the hyper local and non-cultivated vegetables are consumed at least a couple of times every year. • Uphold the culture of special preps during seasons / festivals — undiyo , sarson ka saag during winter, rushi chi bhaji for Ganapati, nadru yakini, etc.	• After the age of five, teach children to have 1 tsp of every vegetable cooked at home. This is a gentle and reasonable way of introducing them to varied tastes without fuss. • Raw and salads are not a part of the Indian food heritage. The only exceptions are kachumbars, raitas and koshimbirs, which are a small part of the meal and not THE meal. • Turning veggies into soup, juices, etc., makes them lose out on all their goodness. • Buy veggies on highways when travelling out for the weekend. Great way to introduce diversity to the diet.
Ghee	• Main meals: A dollop on your roti, rice, paratha, idli, dosa, chilla, khichdi, etc.	• Cook food every day in ghee as per traditional practices and feel free to add more on food while eating.

Food	How to eat	Special notes
	• Mid meals: As a part of homemade laddoos, sheera barfis, halwas, makhana roasted in ghee, roti with ghee and jaggery.	• Homemade ghee made from desi cow milk is the best. If not possible, make from desi buffalo milk. • If homemade ghee is not possible, find a small local dairy or cooperative near you. These days, you will find small goshalas selling ghee online also.
Oils	• Main meals: In cooking, for all sabzis, tadkas, etc. • Mid meals: Use to fry potato, banana, jackfruit, etc. chips at home. • Use it to oil your hair and massage your feet. • Til and coconut oil can be applied / massaged onto the entire body. Especially useful for infants and teens.	• Use the oil local to the region to which you belong. – Ground nut oil: central and western India. – Mustard oil / sesame oil: north and north-east India. – Coconut oil: Kerala. – Many communities use local, non-mainstream seeds for making oil. E.g.: ambadi and native berries in Himalaya. We must preserve this too. • Choose the kacchi ghani oil or cold pressed or filtered or wood-churned oil and not refined / fortified oils.

Food	**How to eat**	**Special notes**
Coconut	• As garnishing on sabzis and dals, as chutney, etc., with main meals. • Nariyal pani, with or without malai, dry coconut and jaggery as a mid-meal.	• If you are into sports, coconut is great for you because of its ability to increase physical stamina and keep your mind calm. • Coconut helps de-stress, so great during exams.
Eggs (if applicable)	• Whole eggs can be eaten every day or as per traditional preferences. • Main meal: Have it with a grain like rice or roti for lunch or dinner. • Mid meal: Can be had just by itself or with a chapatti as an evening snack.	• Buy from a local shop. • Don't remove the egg yolk for the fear of cholesterol. That's outdated news.
Fish, meat (if applicable)	• Can be had three to four days a week or as per traditional practices. • Main meal: Can be had along with a grain like roti or rice. • Should not be eaten as a salad or just with veggies as it can get difficult to digest.	• Buy from a local fish market or butcher shop and avoid the packaged / frozen variety. • Packaged ones are pumped with anti-biotics, chemicals and even steroids, which can come in the way of growth.

Food	How to eat	Special notes
Milk	• Main meal: E.g. shikran poli (roti with banana and milk). • Mid meal: Plain, with or without sugar / with haldi or nuts or fresh fruit or gulkand (in summer) or chyawanprash (in winter). • Can be turned into a homemade traditional sweet like kheer, basundi, sheer kurma during special occasions like Diwali, Eid, etc.	• Buy fresh desi cow or desi buffalo milk from a local dairy. • Avoid Jersey / Holstein cow milk. Avoid Tetra Pak milk. • If you can only drink milk by masking its taste, then don't have it.
Dahi and chaas	• Integral part of the main meal. Gives satiety and works like a digestive aid. • Can be turned into shrikhand (from hung curd). • Khatti chaas into kadhi. • Mid meal: Plain dahi or lassi.	• Home-set dahi from fresh milk and make chaas from it. The best probiotic that you can have. • Set fresh, at least once every day. • Blend using a wooden churner and not an electronic one. • Avoid buying Tetra Pak dahi and chaas.
Makhan / white butter	• Main meal: Can have it with your roti / bhakri / thalipeeth / paratha / kadak pav. • Have it daily or at least weekly.	• This refers to fresh, unsalted white butter made at home.

Food	How to eat	Special notes
Paneer	• Main meal: Sabzi or bhurji with roti or rice. • Mid meal: Sautéed on a tawa with kalanamak and black pepper / paneer mixed with sugar.	• Freshly made at home or bought from a local dairy. • Don't buy the frozen one from the supermarket.
Homemade pickle	• As a small part of the main meal. Makes your meal tasty, improves digestion and the delivery of nutrients to the body, and helps boost immunity. • Combinations like mathri / khakara / puri with homemade aachar make for great mid meal options.	• Should be made using optimum salt, sugar (in case of chunda and murabba), oil (that belongs to your food heritage), and by following the traditional recipes. Don't be scared of using oil and salt — they are crucial to the process of lacto-fermentation. • Store in glass or ceramic containers — no plastic. • Get involved — both boys and girls — in the preparation. • If not possible to make at home, buy from a small cooperative that prepares it fresh, and not branded bottles from the supermarket. • No diet or low fat or low salt or sugar-free versions.

Food	How to eat	Special notes
Papad	• An accompaniment to the main meal • Most papads are better deep fried, some roasted; follow the family tradition.	• Making papad is a great way for the family to bond and spend time together on vacation. • Can also buy from small women's cooperatives. • Dals, veggies, millets — everything is turned into a papad in India. Learn your family's recipe.
Sugar	• WHO recommends no more than six to nine tsp of added sugar daily. If you keep up with traditional eating practices, you won't land up eating more than 2–3 tsp a day. • Main meal: usually a pinch in sabzis, dals and some special preps. • Mid meals: Sherbets, laddoos, halwas, sheera, sugarcane juice, milk, lassi.	• Includes the regular sugar derived from sugarcane. There are people making shakkar the traditional way now, patronise them. • Use the palm, date, coconut sugar if it belongs to your culture and in the specific preparations. • Avoid all sugar substitutes. • Avoid all ultra-processed foods, especially the spreads and dressings. Also juices, colas, chocolates, etc.

Food	How to eat	Special notes
Jaggery	• Mid meal: With roti or in laddoo or chikis, various paaks. • Or just a piece with your main meal.	• In summer — as gud pani. • In winter — as a part of special winter preparations.
Kakvi / molasses	• Mid meal: Along with chapatti, idli, etc.	• Good for anaemia and kidney stones.
Chutneys — made with seeds, nuts, leaves, dals, etc.	• Main meal: Along with your rice and dal or sabzi and roti or khichdi, just like the pickle and papad. • Mid meal: With roti or bhakri / thalipeeth / paratha / dosa / idli / chilla or pudla / upma / dhokla.	• Homemade and traditional: peanut / til / mint / coconut / tomato / garlic / kokum / tamarind, any local variety specific to your region and even household.
Seeds	• Mid meal: Rolled into a laddoo with coconut, ghee and jaggery — great for a school recess dabba. E.g.: aliv seeds. • Can be had soaked in milk during the day. E.g.: sabja. • Can be had as a chutney with chapatti. E.g.: flaxseeds. • Have as a part of mukhwas.	• Various seeds have been used as a part of chutneys, sabzis, sweets, and must be continued to be used as per family traditions. E.g.: charoli in kheers.

Food	How to eat	Special notes
Nuts	• Mid meal: Handful of cashews, almonds, walnuts, pistas, makhana, etc., by themselves, or as part of laddoos and halwas. • Soaked cashews with milk at bedtime to wake up fresh.	• Choose the local and regional variety, e.g., Indian mamra badaam.
Dry fruits	• Mid meal: A handful of dry fruits by themselves or in combination with a nut. E.g., kaju and raisins.	• Can have it first thing on waking up, pre and post games, also during long travels.
Homemade laddoo or barfis or chikis	• Mid meal: As a snack or can be had along with milk for breakfast as well.	• Should be homemade using seasonal ingredients and by following a traditional recipe. • Involve kids when making it at home. • Avoid the packaged ones containing liquid glucose, brown sugar, sweetener or high corn fructose syrup (HFCS).
Homemade dry snacks like chakli, chiwda suhali, etc.	• Great snack for a mid meal anytime during the day.	• Tasty, wholesome and non-perishable. Easy to carry and good option for small breaks or choti bhukh.

Food	How to eat	Special notes
Sherbets	• Can be had daily, especially in summer. Restores electrolyte balance and also rehydrates your body. • Good to have as a mid meal or when playing sports.	• Options you can have include bel sherbet, kokum sherbet, nimbu sherbet, aam panna, khas ka sherbet, variyali sherbet and any other regional one.
Milkshakes	• Mixture of fruit and milk • Mid meal: Between 4 and 6 p.m.	• Make at home, use one fruit only, don't mix many fruits. • Don't add ice cream, chocolates or syrups. • Use fresh milk and not Tetra Pak milk.
Protein powders	• Mix half a scoop in water and have immediately after exercise.	• To be used only by athletes above the age of twelve years. • Go for a whey protein shake which has the least content of added sugar and maximum protein per scoop. (Roughly 25 gm of protein per scoop and less than 1 gm of sugar.)
Gulkand	• Can be had first thing in the morning. • Post your main meals. • Along with milk during the day or at bedtime.	• Can be had all year round, but especially great in summer. • Go for homemade gulkand or buy it from small cooperatives.

Food	How to eat	Special notes
Chyawanprash	• Bedtime or first thing in the morning — one spoonful with milk. • Daily during winter.	• Help your dadi or nani make it along with all your cousins and friends. • Avoid mass-produced ones. Buy it from someone who makes it fresh at home or from small organisations.
Homemade samosa, bhajiya kachori, etc.	• Once a week. Or on festivals like Diwali, Dussehra, Eid, Rakshabandhan, etc. • Daily, during winter.	• Go for the proper deep fried ones and not air fried or baked. • And please use traditional ground nut or mustard oil for frying.
Muramba / homemade jams	• Mid meal: With roti or bread.	• Made with seasonal fruits, berries, etc., add diverse nutrient profile and should be preferred over packaged and processed ones.
Honey	• Used as medicine for sore throat, cold and cough.	• Look for freshly collected wild honey and not the packaged one in malls. • Buy from tribals, small and government-backed cooperatives.

Group 2: Foods you should not eat more than once a month

Surprise! This list is much shorter than the one above. Goes to prove the variety and diversity available in our kitchens that will beat these processed / packaged foods and drinks hollow any day — on taste, nourishment and satiety. Not to mention, these foods fail all the three tests, don't support local economies and damage the environment. Limit them to once a month, max. So one or two of these items, once a month, if you must.

Foods	How to eat	Special notes
Biscuits, breads and cereals	• Can be had as mid meals and not as main meals.	• Choose from a local bakery instead of buying the packaged, processed type. • Contain GRAS and designer food molecules which keep you addicted to them and that's why you end up craving them frequently.*
Chocolates, brownies, ice creams and cupcakes	• Mid meal: Can be had between 4 and 6 p.m. • Don't have post dinner.	• Affects growth and causes dehydration. Often contain artificial colours and flavours. • If homemade, limit the quantity and frequency of making them.

* This is common for all the foods in this table.

Foods	How to eat	Special notes
		• Know that chocolate industries employ child labour and there is almost no way to know for sure if the chocolate you are eating was ethically grown.
World cuisines like Chinese, Korean, Italian, Mexican, Thai	• Can be had daily if you are travelling in that country.	• Eat fresh out of a gourmet restaurant and not a fast food joint which promises 'thirty-minute delivery'. • Go for only one type of cuisine in one meal, preferably the one that is local to that region.
Chaat	• Pani puri, sev puri, dahi puri, dahi bada, ragada pattice, pav bhaji and the likes. • Can be planned as an evening meal between 4 and 6 p.m. Never to be had as lunch or dinner.	• Have only one type of chaat at a time. • Choose the one that you like the most. • Local, street food typically doesn't have GRAS or designer food molecules.
Ready-to-eat stuff that gets cooked / fried in two to five minutes — instant noodles, pasta, fries, etc.	• Can be had as a mid meal, never as a main meal.	• Zero in nutrients even though they claim to be fortified with vitamins. In fact, they slow down growth.

Foods	How to eat	Special notes
		• All varieties are equally bad. You may pay more for those considered healthier — the ones with oats / veggies, etc. — but they are not better. • Surely not to be packed in tiffin or served at birthday parties.
Ketchups, sauces, spreads and salad dressings	• You can use chutneys in your sandwich instead.	• Very low on nutrients, contain sweeteners, artificial flavours and colours.
Packaged cheese	• Mid meal: Just by itself in the form of a cube or a slice or with bread or roti and chutney. • Cheese as part of your pasta or pizza or any other dish — once a month.	• Handy to eat while travelling. • Don't confuse this with local, fresh cheese like paneer, which you could have more often. You can even buy fresh cheese while on trips abroad from farmers' markets, but get small quantities.
Packaged butter	• On bread or on pav when eating pav bhaji.	• Yellow, salted or unsalted or any flavour — of any brand.
Peanut butter and nut butters	• Mid meal: On bread or a cracker or a sandwich.	• Made using refined vegetable oils, and poor grade salt and sugar.

Foods	How to eat	Special notes
Palm oil or edible vegetable oil	• Most often found in biscuits, packaged popcorn, chips, spreads, pizzas.	• Palm oil is cheap as it is subsidised by many countries, including ours. • Palm cultivation is quite ecologically unsustainable.
Sweeteners / sugar substitutes like stevia and sugars like HFCS	• Present in packaged / processed products like cereals, biscuits, etc. • Also juices, colas, chocolates, cakes, etc.	• Sweeteners are generally used as alternatives to sugar in sugar-free products. Instead of being healthier, they make our brains slow and dull, and our bones weak. • This is the stuff you should be avoiding, not the homemade laddoos and halwas.
Popcorn	• Eat roasted or boiled native varieties, instead of popcorn. • Native or local corn come in a variety of colours — white to deep orange and even purple.	• Marketed as the must-eat food in movie theatres, packaged popcorn is poor on nutrients. • Market currently flooded with the American one or sweet corn. Demand local, native species.
Chips and wafers	• Mid meal or snack.	• Buy from a local, small shop which makes them fresh and in small quantities.

Foods	How to eat	Special notes
		• The ultra-processed chips not only damage the inside of your body, but the outside environment too.
Juices, smoothies, colas and caffeinated energy drinks	• Fresh sugarcane juice is an exception; it can be had once every day (in season) up to 4 p.m.	• Packaged juices contain preservatives, artificial flavours, excess sugar of poor quality. • Even if you make it fresh and at home, this is not a traditional practice and fruits should be eaten whole. • Avoid readymade shakes. • Caffeine drinks and colas are very high on poor quality sugar and also deplete underground water resources. • Buy in small glass bottles and not big family packs
Chai / coffee	• Athletes, especially, should avoid both. • Even milky teas and coffees are to be avoided by kids.	• Tea contains an anti-nutrient called tannin and coffee contains an anti-nutrient called caffeine — these come in the way of calcium and iron absorption, which comes in the way of growth and good skin and most importantly good sleep (in case of caffeine).

Foods	How to eat	Special notes
		• Don't have them to stay up during exams — dry coconut and jaggery is a much healthier alternative.
Flavoured powders to be added to milk and nut milks	• Drinking milk is not compulsory for calcium or protein. • These are not a substitute to drinking milk.	• If you can only drink milk by adding these powders, it's better to not have milk. • Also, nut milks are being produced in an ecologically insensitive way due to huge demands after its positioning as a better alternative to milk.
Packaged water	• Avoid as far as possible. • Best to carry your own steel bottle and refill it with local water of the region. Supports the gut microbes and allows you to adjust to the local food of the place.	• Drink local water — filter and boil if unsure of the source / purity. • Single-use plastic, whether for water or colas, etc., must be avoided. • Costly ecologically — takes up huge amounts of ground water.